CW00502346

Delicious Veggie Recipes

A Complete Collection of Tasty Vegetarian Recipes for Your Daily Lunch & Dinner

Kaylee Collins

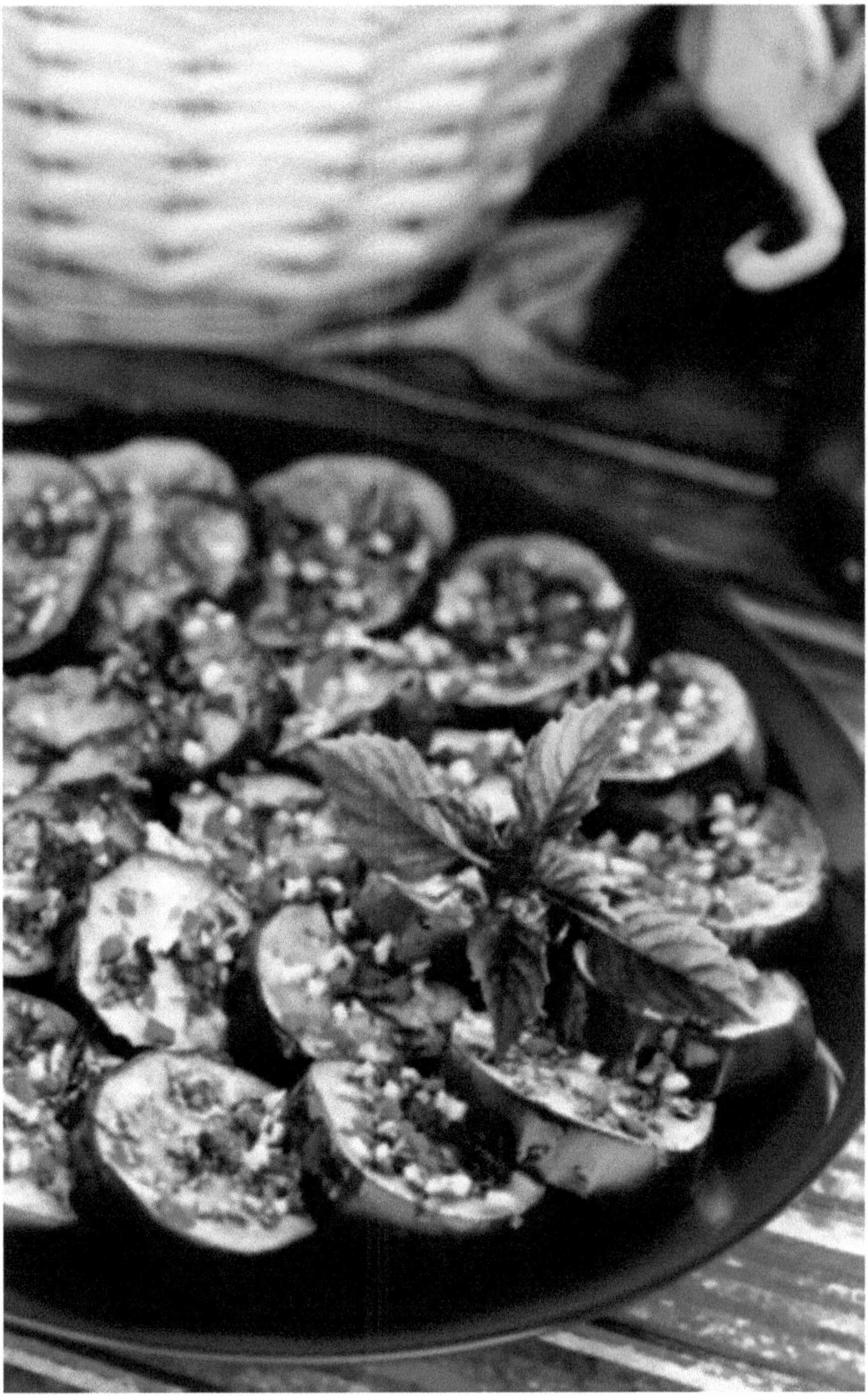

By reading this document, the reader agrees that under no circumstances is the author responsible for any losses, direct or indirect, which are incurred as a result of the use of information contained within this document, including, but not limited to, — errors, omissions, or inaccuracies.

Table of Contents

6

Baked Watercress and Summer Squash

Ingredients

1 ½ pounds summer squash, peeled and cut into 1-inch chunks

½ red onion, thinly sliced

¼ cup water

½ vegetable stock cube, crumbled

1 tbsp. sesame oil

½ tsp Chinese

5 spice powder

½ tsp Sichuan Peppercorns

½ tsp hot chili powder

Black pepper

½ pound fresh watercress, roughly chopped

Directions:

Put all of the ingredients in a slow cooker except the last one. Top with handfuls of watercress and stuff the slow cooker with it. If you can't fit it all in at once, let the first batch cook first and add some more watercress. Cook for 3 or 4 hours on medium until summer squash becomes soft. Scrape the sides and serve.

Curried Kale and Rutabaga

Ingredients

1 ½ pound Rutabaga, peeled and cut into 1-inch chunks

½ onion, thinly sliced

¼ cup water

½ vegetable stock cube, crumbled

1 tbsp. extra virgin olive oil

½ tsp cumin

½ tsp ground coriander

½ tsp garam masala

½ tsp hot chili powder Black pepper

½ pound fresh kale, roughly chopped

Directions:

Put all of the ingredients in a slow cooker except the last one. Top with handfuls of kale and stuff the slow cooker with it. If you can't fit it all in at once, let the first batch cook first and add some more kale. Cook for 3or 4 hours on medium until root vegetables become soft. Scrape the sides and serve

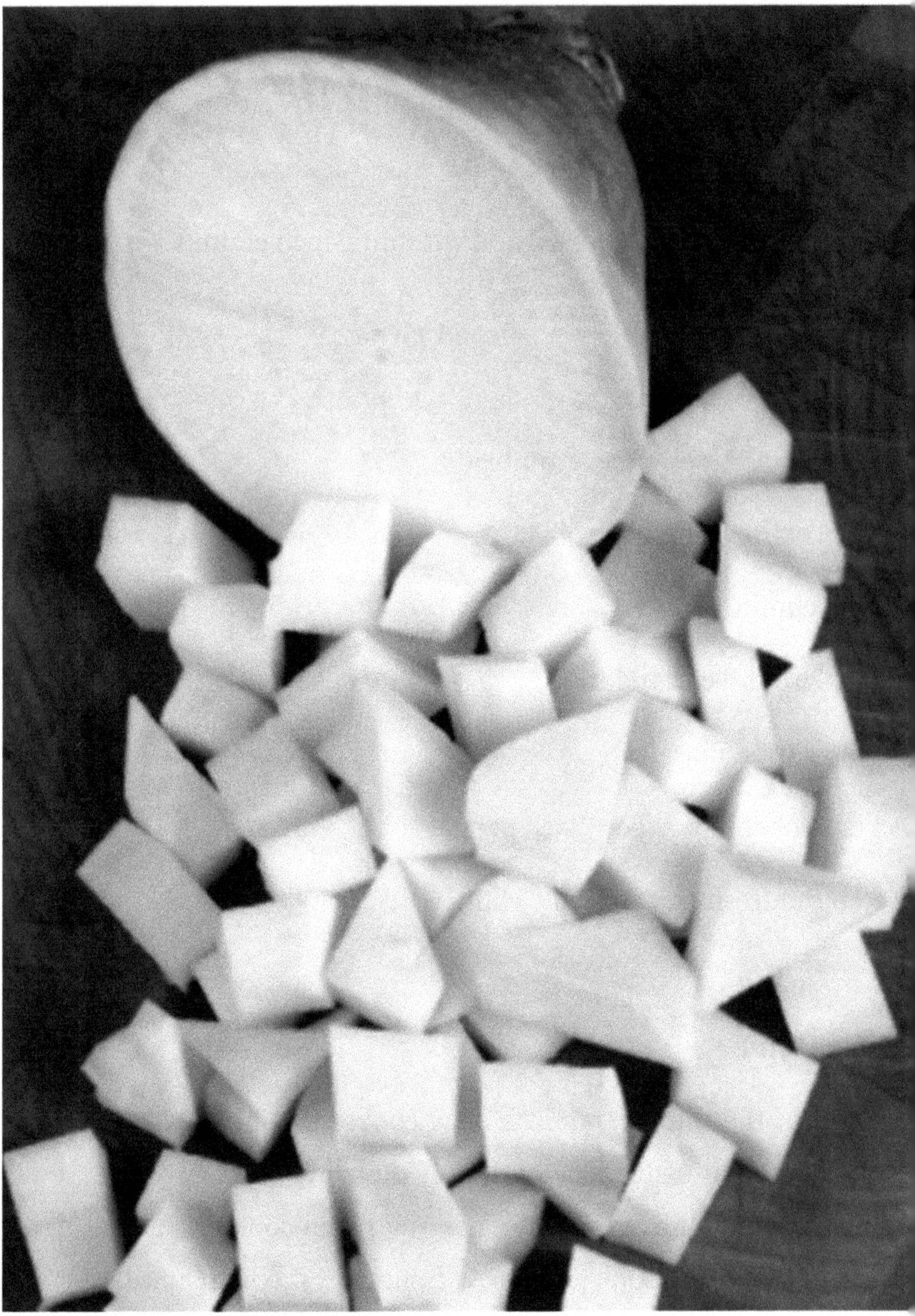

Buttered Potatoes and Spinach

Ingredients

1 ½ pounds red potatoes, peeled and cut into 1-inch chunks

½ onion, thinly sliced

¼ cup water

½ vegetable stock cube, crumbled

2 tbsp. salted butter

½ tsp herbs de Provence

½ tsp thyme

½ tsp hot chili powder

Black pepper

½ pound fresh spinach, roughly chopped

Directions:

Put all of the ingredients in a slow cooker except the last one. Top with handfuls of spinach and stuff the slow cooker with it. If you can't fit it all in at once, let the first batch cook first and add some more spinach. Cook for 3or 4 hours on medium until potatoes become soft. Scrape the sides and serve.

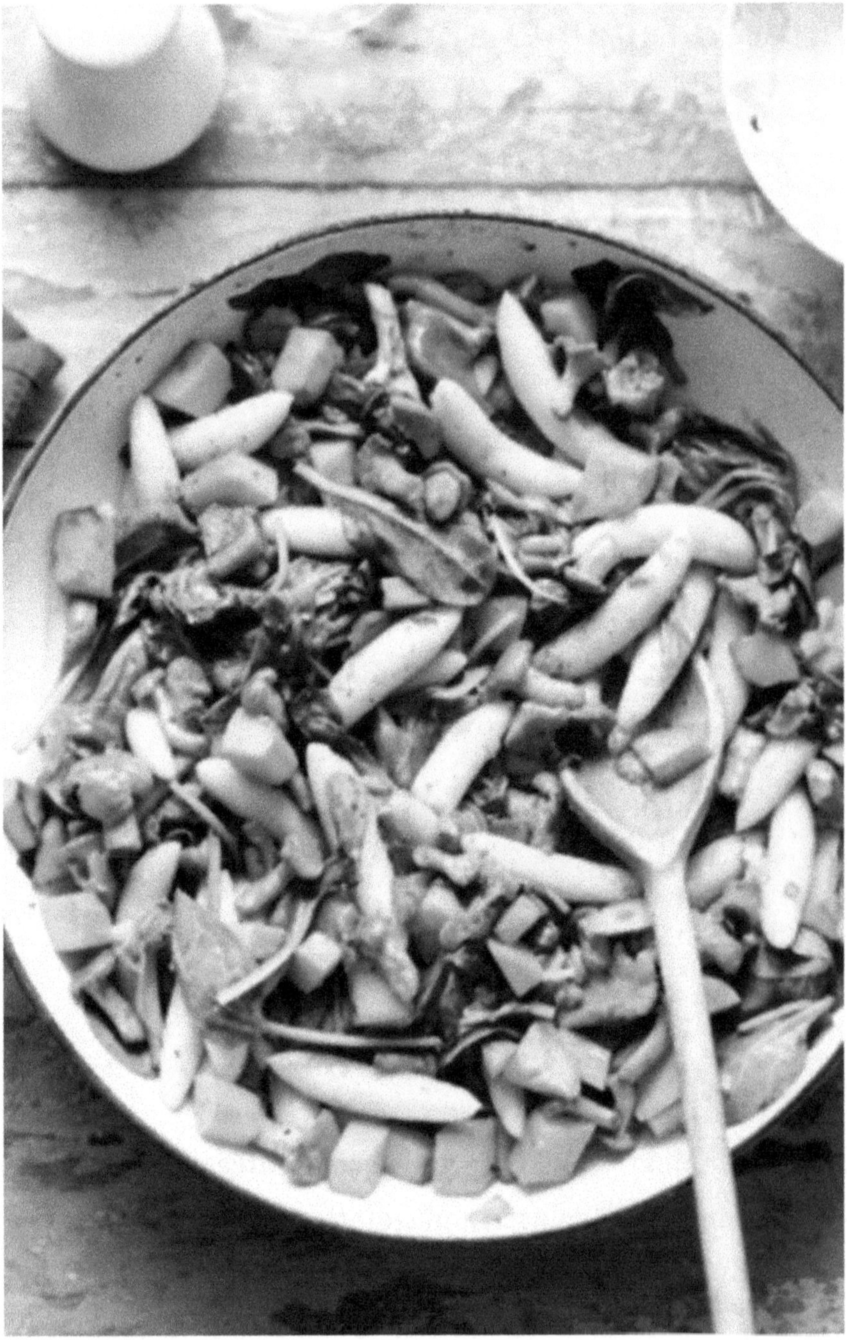

Roasted Vegan-Buttered Mustard Greens Carrots

Ingredients

1 ½ pounds carrots, peeled and cut into 1-inch chunks ½ onion, thinly sliced

¼ cup water

½ vegetable stock cube, crumbled

1 tbsp. butter

1 tsp garlic, minced

½ tsp lemon juice

Black pepper

½ pound fresh mustard greens, roughly chopped

Directions:

Put all of the ingredients in a slow cooker except the last one. Top with handfuls of mustard greens and stuff the slow cooker with it. If you can't fit it all in at once, let the first batch cook first and add some more mustard greens. Cook for 3or 4 hours on medium until carrots become soft. Scrape the sides and serve.

Smoky Roasted Swiss Chard and Cauliflower

Ingredients

1 ½ pounds cauliflower, peeled and cut into 1-inch chunks

½ red onion, thinly sliced

¼ cup water

½ vegetable stock cube, crumbled

1 tbsp. extra virgin olive oil

½ tsp cumin

½ tsp hot chili powder

Black pepper

½ pound fresh Swiss chard, roughly chopped

Directions:

Put all of the ingredients in a slow cooker except the last one. Top with handfuls of Swiss chard and stuff the slow cooker with it. If you can't fit it all in at once, let the first batch cook first and add some more Swiss chard. Cook for 3or 4 hours on medium until potatoes become soft. Scrape the sides and serve.

Roasted Microgreens and Potatoes

Ingredients

1 ½ pounds potatoes, peeled and cut into 1-inch chunks ½ onion, thinly sliced

¼ cup water

½ vegetable stock cube, crumbled

1 tbsp. olive oil

½ tsp minced ginger

2 sprigs of lemon grass

½ tsp green onions, minced

½ tsp hot chili powder

Black pepper

½ pound Microgreens, roughly chopped

Directions:

Put all of the ingredients in a slow cooker except the last one. Top with handfuls of Microgreens and stuff the slow cooker with it. If you can't fit it all in at once, let the first batch cook first and add some more Microgreens. Cook for 3or 4 hours on medium until potatoes become soft. Scrape the sides and serve.

Roasted Spinach & Broccoli with Jalapeno

Ingredients

1 ½ pound broccoli florets

½ onion, thinly sliced

¼ cup water

½ vegetable stock cube, crumbled

1 tbsp. extra virgin olive oil

½ tsp cumin

8 jalapeno peppers, finely chopped

1 ancho chili

½ tsp hot chili powder

Black pepper

½ pound fresh spinach, roughly chopped

Directions:

Put all of the ingredients in a slow cooker except the last one. Top with handfuls of spinach and stuff the slow cooker with it. If you can't fit it all in at once, let the first batch cook first and add some more spinach. Cook for 3or 4 hours on medium until broccoli becomes soft. Scrape the sides and serve.

Spicy Baked Swiss Chard and Cauliflower

Ingredients

1 ½ pound cauliflower florets, blanched (dipped in boiling water then dipped in ice water)

½ cup bean sprouts, rinsed

½ cup water

½ vegetable stock cube, crumbled

1 tbsp. sesame oil

½ tsp Thai chili paste

½ tsp Sriracha hot sauce

½ tsp hot chili powder

2 Thai bird chilies, minced Black pepper

½ pound fresh Swiss chard, roughly chopped

Directions:

Put all of the ingredients in a slow cooker except the last one. Top with handfuls of Swiss chard and stuff the slow cooker with it. If you can't fit it all in at once, let the first batch cook first and add some more Swiss chard. Cook for 3 or 4 hours on medium until potatoes become soft. Scrape the sides and serve.

Thai Carrots and Collard Greens

Ingredients

1 ½ pounds carrots, peeled and cut into 1-inch chunks ½ onion, thinly sliced

¼ cup water

½ vegetable stock cube, crumbled

1 tbsp. extra virgin olive oil

1 tbsp. sesame oil

½ tsp Thai chili paste

½ tsp Sriracha hot sauce

½ tsp hot chili powder

2 Thai bird chilies, minced Black pepper

½ pound collard greens, roughly chopped

Directions:

Put all of the ingredients in a slow cooker except the last one. Top with handfuls of collard greens and stuff the slow cooker with it. If you can't fit it all in at once, let the first batch cook first and add some more collard greens. Cook for 3or 4 hours on medium until carrots become soft. Scrape the sides and serve.

Baked White Yam and Spinach

Ingredients

½ pounds potatoes, peeled and cut into 1-inch chunks ½ pounds white yam, peeled and cut into 1-inch chunks ½ pounds carrots, peeled and cut into 1- inch chunks

½ red onion, thinly sliced

¼ cup water

½ vegetable stock cube, crumbled

1 tbsp. extra virgin olive oil

½ tsp cumin

½ tsp ground coriander

½ tsp garam masala

½ tsp cayenne pepper Black pepper

½ pound fresh spinach, roughly chopped

Directions:

Put all of the ingredients in a slow cooker except the last one. Top with handfuls of spinach and stuff the slow cooker with it. If you can't fit it all in at once, let the first batch cook first and add some more spinach. Cook for 3or 4 hours on medium until potatoes become soft. Scrape the sides and serve.

Southeast Asian Baked Turnip Greens & Carrots

Ingredients

½ pound turnips, peeled and cut into 1-inch chunks

½ pound carrots, peeled and cut into 1-inch chunks

½ pound parsnips, peeled and cut into 1-inch chunks

½ red onion, thinly sliced

½ cup vegetable broth

1 tbsp. extra virgin olive oil

½ tsp minced ginger

2 stalks lemon grass

8 cloves garlic, minced

Black pepper

½ pound fresh turnip greens, roughly chopped

Directions:

Put all of the ingredients in a slow cooker except the last one. Top with handfuls of turnip greens and stuff the slow cooker with it. If you can't fit it all in at once, let the first batch cook first and add some more turnip greens. Cook for 3or 4 hours on medium until turnips become soft. Scrape the sides and serve.

Curried Watercress and Potatoes

Ingredients

1 ½ pounds potatoes, peeled and cut into 1-inch chunks ½ onion, thinly sliced

¼ cup water

½ vegetable stock cube, crumbled

1 tbsp. extra virgin olive oil

½ tsp cumin

½ tsp ground coriander

½ tsp garam masala

½ tsp hot chili powder

Black pepper

½ pound fresh Watercress, roughly chopped

Directions:

Put all of the ingredients in a slow cooker except the last one. Top with handfuls of watercress and stuff the slow cooker with it. If you can't fit it all in at once, let the first batch cook first and add some more watercress. Cook for 3or 4 hours on medium until potatoes become soft. Scrape the sides and serve.

Jalapeno Kale and Parsnips

Ingredients

1 ½ pounds parsnips, peeled and cut into

1-inch chunks

½ red onion, thinly sliced

¼ cup water

½ vegetable stock cube, crumbled

1 tbsp. extra virgin olive oil

½ tsp cumin

½ tsp jalapeno pepper, minced

1 ancho chili, minced Black pepper

½ pound Kale, roughly chopped

Directions:

Put all of the ingredients in a slow cooker except the last one. Top with handfuls of kale and stuff the slow cooker with it. If you can't fit it all in at once, let the first batch cook first and add some more Kale. Cook for 3or 4 hours on medium until parsnips become soft. Scrape the sides and serve.

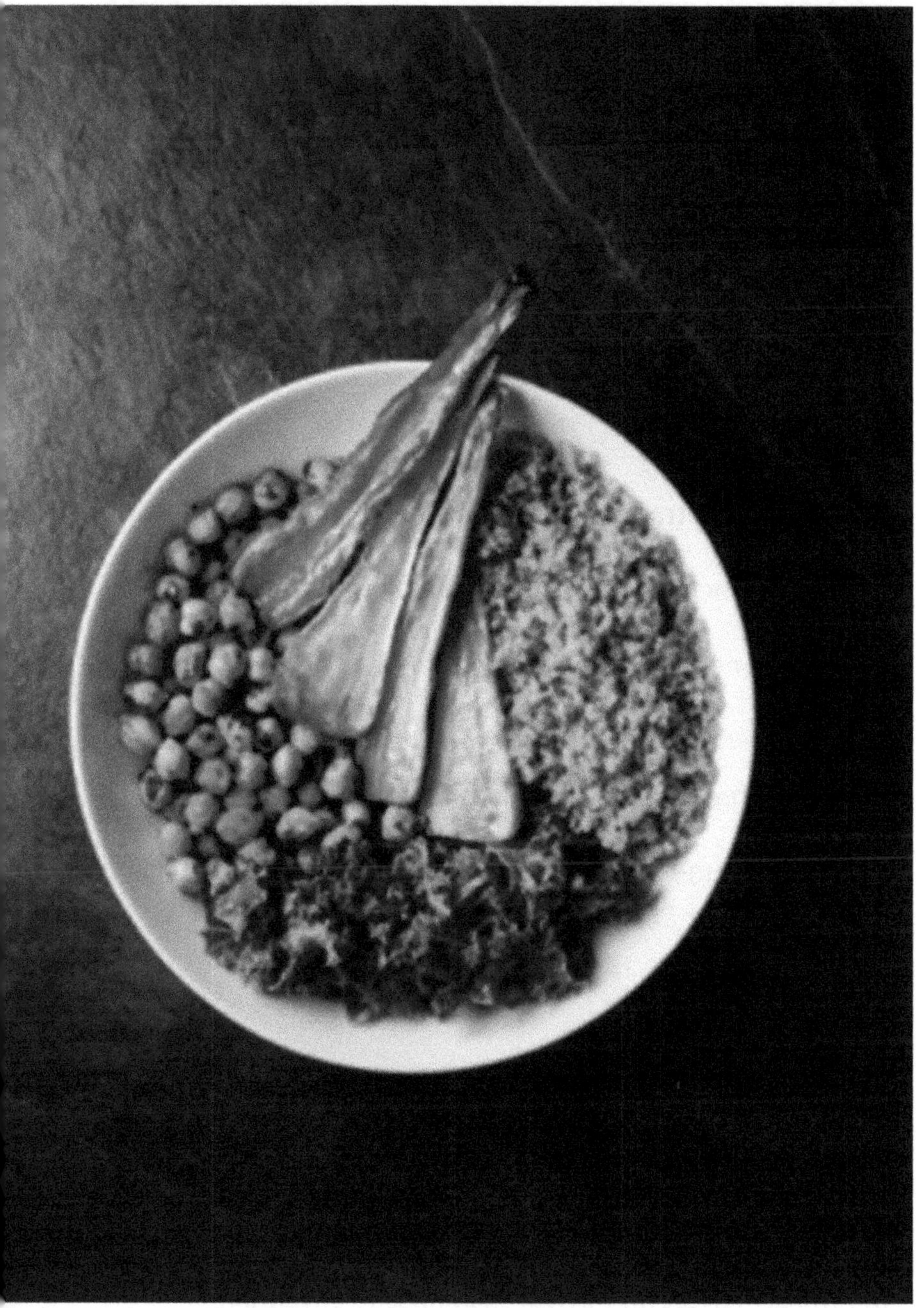

Spinach and Zucchini Lasagna Recipe

Prep Time: 20 minutes Cook Time: 50 minutes

Total Time: 1 hour 10 minutes

Servings: 9 people

Ingredients

1 tablespoon extra virgin olive oil

½ onion - finely chopped 4 garlic cloves - crushed

1 tablespoons tomato paste

1 28-ounce can crushed tomatoes with the juice or 1¾ pounds of fresh tomatoes - peeled, seeded, and diced

Salt and ground fresh black pepper to taste 1 tablespoon fresh basil - chopped

3 cups spinach

15 ounces part-skim ricotta 1 large egg

½ cup freshly grated Parmesan cheese

4 medium zucchini - sliced ⅛-inch thick

16 ounces part-skim mozzarella cheese - shredded

½ teaspoon parsley - chopped

Instructions

In a saucepan, heat the olive oil over medium heat.

Add the onions, and cook 4-5 minutes until they are soft and golden. Add the garlic, and sauté, being careful not to burn the garlic. Add the tomato paste and stir well. Add the chopped tomatoes, including the juice in case you are using canned tomatoes. Add salt and ground fresh black pepper. Bring to a low simmer, cover, and cook for 25-30 minutes. Finally, remove from the heat, and add the fresh basil and spinach. Stir well. Adjust the seasoning if necessary. Arrange the zucchini slices in a single layer on a baking sheet coated with cooking oil spray. Broil for 5-8 minutes. Remove from the oven. Wait about 5 minutes to remove any excess moisture with paper towels if necessary. (This part is very important to avoid the lasagna becoming too soupy.) Preheat the oven to 375°F.

In a medium bowl, mix the ricotta cheese, Parmesan cheese, and egg. Stir well.

In a 9x12-inch casserole, spread some tomato-spinach sauce on the bottom. Layer 5 or 6 zucchini slices to cover. Place some of the ricotta cheese mixture on the zucchini slices, and top with some mozzarella cheese. Repeat the layers until all your ingredients are used. Top with sauce and mozzarella. Cover the casserole dish with aluminum foil, and bake for 30 minutes. Uncover, and cook an additional 10-15 minutes. Let stand about 10 minutes before serving. Garnish with parsley.

Nutrition Info

Calories: 223kcal Carbohydrates: 10.6g Protein: 18.5g

Fat: 12.4g Cholesterol: 53mg Sugar: 4.4g

Vegan Sesame Tofu and Eggplant

Servings 4

Ingredients

1 pound firm tofu, block

1 cup fresh cilantro, chopped, ~31g

3 tablespoons unseasoned rice vinegar 4 tablespoons toasted sesame oil

2 cloves garlic, finely minced

1 teaspoon crushed red pepper flakes 2 teaspoons Swerve confectioners

1 whole eggplant, ~458g 1 tablespoon olive oil Salt and pepper to taste

¼ cup sesame seeds

¼ cup soy sauce

Instructions

Preheat oven to 200°F. Remove the block of tofu from it's packaging and wrap with some paper towels. Place a plate on top of it and weigh it down. I used a really large tin of vegetables in this picture, but you can use anything handy. Let the tofu sit for a while to press some of the water out. Place about ¼ cup of cilantro, 3 tablespoons rice vinegar, 2 tablespoons toasted sesame oil, minced garlic, crushed red pepper flakes, and Swerve into a large mixing bowl. Whisk together. Peel and julienne the eggplant. You can julienne roughly by hand like I did, or use a mandolin with a julienne attachment for more precise "noodles." Mix the eggplant with the marinade. Add the tablespoon of olive oil to a skillet over medium-low heat. Cook the eggplant until it softens. The eggplant will soak up all of the li☐uids, so if you have issues with it sticking to the pan, feel free to add a little bit more sesame or olive oil. Just be sure to adjust your Nutrition Info tracking.

Turn the oven off. Stir the remaining cilantro into the eggplant then transfer the noodles to an oven safe dish. Cover with a lid, or foil, and place into the oven to keep warm. Wipe out the skillet and return to the stovetop to heat up again. Unwrap the tofu then cut into 8 slices. Spread the sesame seeds on a plate. Press both sides of each piece of tofu into the seeds. Add 2 tablespoons of sesame oil to the skillet. Fry both sides of the tofu for 5 minutes each, or until they start to crisp up. Pour the ¼ cup of soy sauce into the pan and coat the pieces of tofu. Cook until the tofu slices look browned and caramelized with the soy sauce.

Remove the noodles from the oven and plate the tofu on top.

Nutrition Info

292.75 Calories 24.45g Fats 6.87g Net Carbs 11.21g Protein.

Keto Pierogies Using Fathead Dough

Delicious Keto Pierogies made with Fathead Dough are the perfect low carb pierogi substitute! You can fill them with almost anything but this version uses cheesy cauliflower puree!

Prep Time: 20 minutes Cook Time: 17 minutes Total Time: 37 minutes Servings: 12

Ingredients

For the Keto Pierogi Dough:

2 cups super fine blanched almond flour

2 cups shredded full fat mozzarella cheese 1/4 cup butter

1 large egg

1 large egg yolk For the Keto Pierogi Filling:

1 cup Cheesy Cauliflower Puree, chilled or at room temperature 1 tsp dried onion flakes

To cook and serve:

1/2 cup thinly sliced yellow onions 3 Tbsp butter

salt and pepper to taste

Instructions

To make the Keto Pierogi Dough:

Combine the mozzarella cheese and butter in a medium bowl and microwave for 1 minute. Stir, then microwave another minute. Stir until fully combined and cool for 2 minutes. Stir in the egg and egg yolk until combined.

Add the almond flour and stir with a large spoon until combined. Turn out dough onto smooth surface (or parchment paper) and knead until a semi-stretchy dough is formed. (if the dough is too wet, add a tablespoon or more of almond flour until workable)

To make the Keto Pierogies:

Divide the dough into 12 equally sized balls. Press each ball into a disk about 4 inches around.

Combine the Cheesy Cauliflower Puree and dried onion flakes and mix well. Place about 1.5 tablespoons of room temperature Cheesy Cauliflower Puree onto one half of each disk, leaving a half inch border to seal. Fold the dough over the filling and pinch to seal. Chill 10 minutes or freeze until ready to use (if cooking from frozen, thaw first).

To cook and serve the Keto Pierogi:

Melt the butter in a large saute pan over medium heat.

Add the onions and cook for 5 minutes or until soft and translucent. Add 6 of the pierogies to the pan and cook for 3 minutes per side or until the dough has turned golden brown. Remove and set aside.

Cook the remaining 6 pierogies the same way. Serve warm with the onions and butter over the top.

Nutrition Info

Serving Size: 2 Pierogies with 1 Tbsp onions in butter Calories: 503

Fat: 46g Carbohydrates: 7g net Protein: 20g

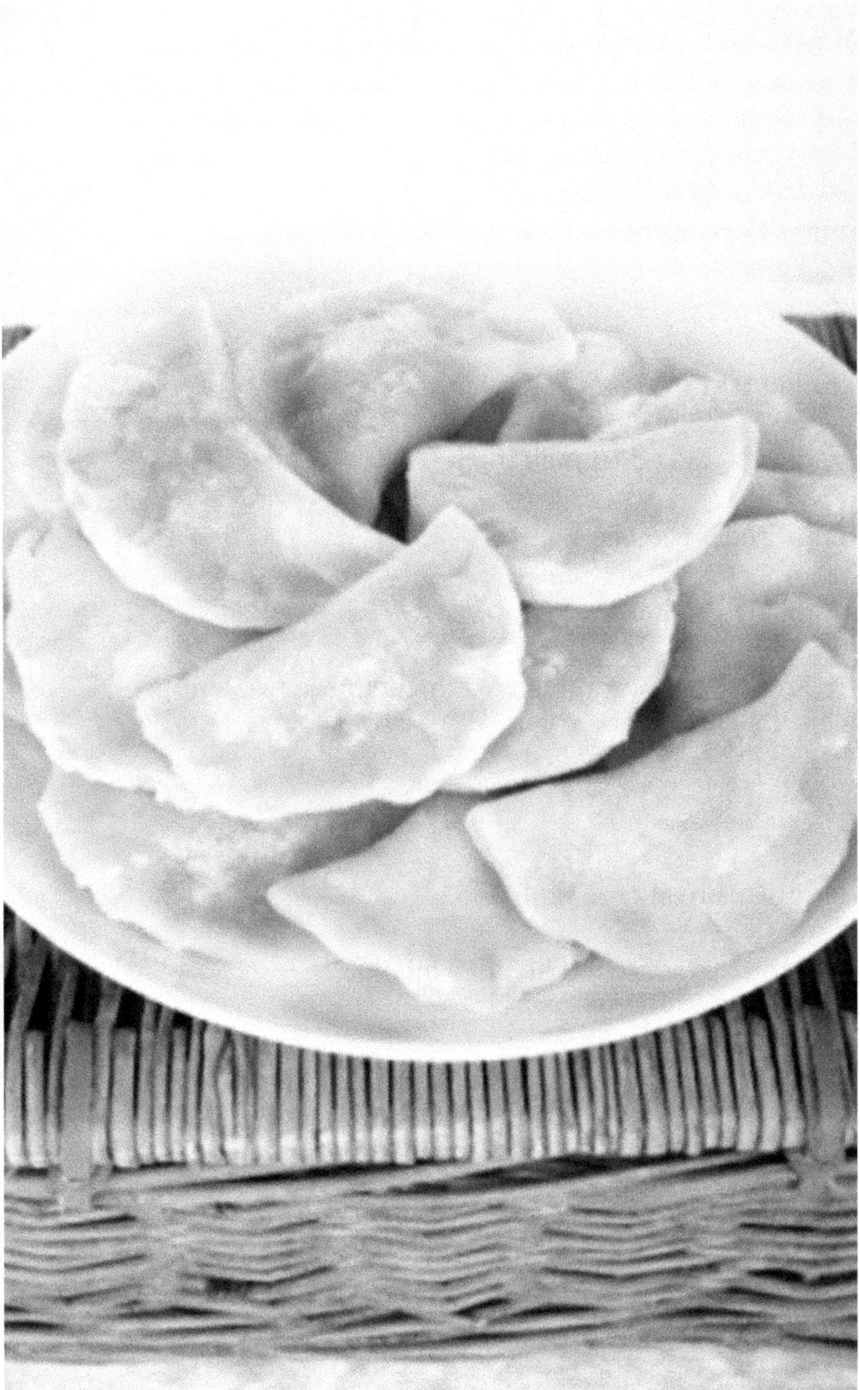

Eggplant Gratin With Feta Cheese

Prep Time: 15 minutes Cook Time: 40 minutes Total Time: 55 minutes Servings: 6

Ingredients

2 eggplants , sliced ½ inch thick

½ cup Crème Fraîche

½ cup half and half

3 oz Feta cheese crumbled 1 tsp thyme leaves chopped 1 tbsp chives chopes

4-5 basil leaves

¾ cup Gruyere cheese grated

½ cup tomato sauce 3 tbsp olive oil

salt, pepper to taste

Instructions

Preheat the oven to 375 F.

Place sliced eggplant on a parchment lined baking pan (you might need to use 2 pans). Sprinkle both sides with salt and pepper and brush with olive oil. Bake for about 20 minutes until eggplant is tender. Meanwhile, in a small saucepan, combine Crème fraîche, half and half and Feta cheese. Bring to a boil and remove from the heat. Stir in thyme and chives and set aside.

In 2.5-☐uart baking dish or gratin dish spread tomato sauce to cover the bottom. Place eggplant slices. They can slightly overlap each other. Spread tomato sauce once again and sprinkle with ¼ cup of Gruyere cheese. Scatter 1-2 torn basil leaves over the sauce. Continue layering with remaining eggplant, sauce and basil. Finish with pouring over the cream and Feta sauce and sprinkling with the remaining Gruyere cheese.

Bake for 15-20 minutes until bubbly and the top is browned. Serve warm.

Nutrition Info

Calories: 302kcal Carbohydrates: 14g Protein: 9.4g

Fat: 24.3g

Saturated Fat: 11.7g Cholesterol: 34mg Sodium: 335mg Potassium: 534mg Fiber: 6.8g

Sugar: 7.7g

Calcium: 220mg

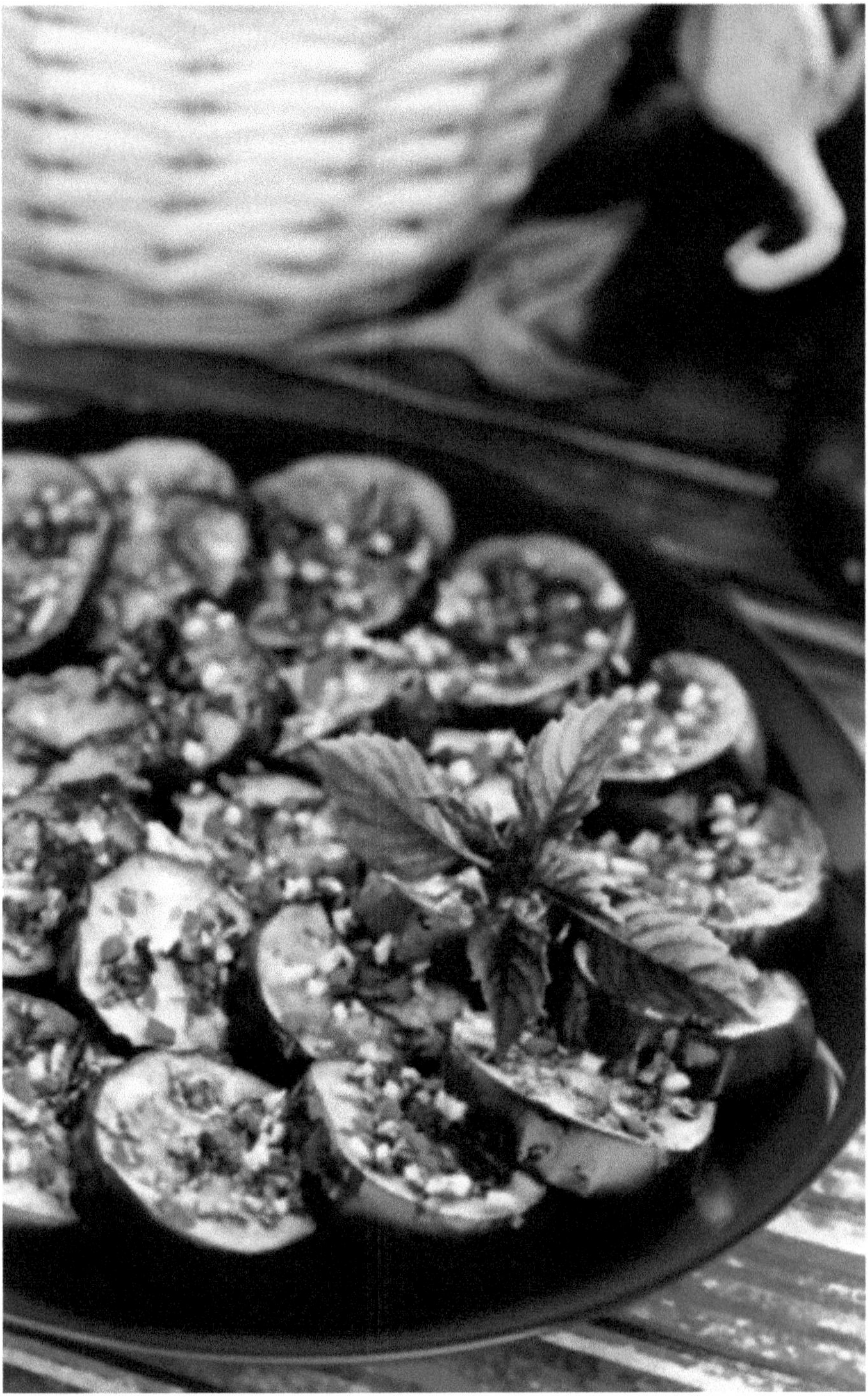

Roasted Caprese Tomatoes with Basil dressing

Roasted Caprese tomatoes with creamy mozzarella and fresh basil is a delicious and easy side dish recipe and perfect as a Summer appetizer served with crusty bread.

Prep Time: 5 minutes Cook Time: 30 minutes Total Time: 35 minutes Servings: 4

Ingredients

6 ripe tomatoes

1 tablespoon olive oil

2 tablespoons Balsamic vinegar salt & pepper to taste

6 thin slices Mozzarella 6 basil leaves for the dressing

small handful fresh basil 1 garlic clove

juice of 1/2 lemon

2 tablespoons olive oil salt and pepper to taste

Instructions

Pre-heat the oven to 180°C/350°F.

Halve the tomatoes and place on a non-stick baking sheet, cut side up. Drizzle over the olive oil and Balsamic and season with salt and pepper then top the 4 bottom halves with the mozzarella and basil leaves. Add the tops of the tomatoes. Roast for 20-25 minutes until the skins are blistered and the tomatoes are soft.

To make the dressing, blitz all the ingredients in a small food processor until the basil is finely chopped. Serve the tomatoes drizzled with the dressing with crusty bread.

Nutrition Info

Calories: 198kcal Carbohydrates: 9g Protein: 8g

Fat: 15g Saturated Fat: 4g

Cholesterol: 16mg Sodium: 166mg Potassium: 467mg Fiber: 2g

Sugar: 6g

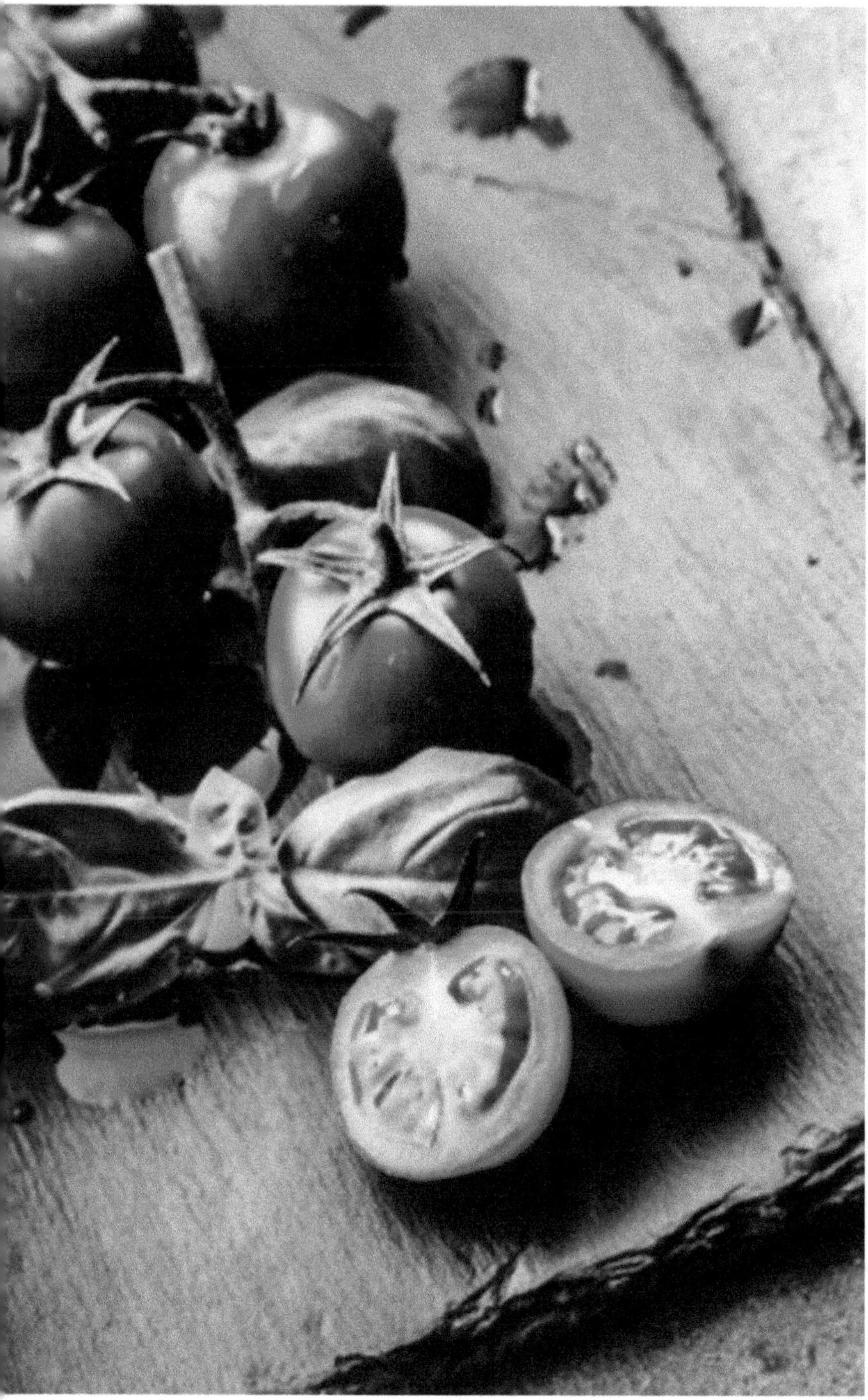

Cheesy Low Carb Cauliflower Risotto in Creamy Pesto Sauce

This versatile low carb side dish recipe perfectly mimics a classic risotto but is made with cauliflower and smothered in a cheesy pesto sauce. Keto and Atkins friendly.

Servings: Four 1 cup serving

Ingredients

4 cups finely chopped (or grated) raw cauliflower 2 Tbsp butter

1/2 tsp kosher salt 1/8 tsp black pepper 1/4 tsp garlic powder

1/3 cup Mascarpone cheese 2 Tbsp Parmesan cheese 1/4 cup prepared basil pesto

Instructions

Combine the cauliflower, butter, salt, pepper, and garlic powder in a microwave safe bowl. Microwave on high for six minutes – or until the cauliflower is tender and done to your liking. Add the mascarpone cheese and microwave on high for 2 more minutes.

Add the parmesan cheese and stir until fully blended and creamy. Cool for 2 minutes (so you don't cook the pesto when you add it and lose the green color.)

Stir in the basil pesto and serve warm.

Nutrition Info

225 calories 21g fat

4g net carbs 6g protein

Vegetarian Greek Collard Wraps

Servingss 4 servings

Ingredients

Tzatziki Sauce

1 cup full-fat plain Greek yogurt 1 teaspoon garlic powder

1 tablespoon white vinegar 2 tablespoons olive oil

2.5 ounces cucumber, seeded and grated (¼-whole) 2 tablespoons minced fresh dill

Salt and pepper to taste

The Wrap

4 large collard green leaves, washed

1 medium cucumber, julienned

½ medium red bell pepper, julienned

½ cup purple onion, diced

8 whole kalamata olives, halved

½ block feta, cut into 4 (1-inch thick) strips (4-oz) 4 large cherry tomatoes, halved

Instructions

Mix all of the ingredients for the tzatziki sauce together and also store in the fridge. Be sure to s☐ueeze all of the water out of the cucumber after you grate it. Prepare collard green wraps by washing leaves well and trimming the fibrous stem from each leaf. Spread 2 tablespoons of tzatziki onto the center of each wrap and smooth the sauce out. Layer the cucumber, pepper, onion, olives, feta and tomatoes in the center of the wrap. I've shown them spread out in a line to display each ingredient, but when assembling these wraps it works best to keep all of the ingredients close and toward the center of the leaf. Imagine piling them high rather than spreading them out! Fold as you would a burrito, folding in each side toward the center and the folding the rounded end over the filling and roll. Slice in halves and serve with any leftover tzatziki or wrap in plastic for a quick lunchtime meal!

Nutrition Info

165.34 Calories

11.25 g Fat 7.36g Net Carbs 6.98g Protein

Red Cabbage Coleslaw

Ingredients

¼ of a large red cabbage, shredded with a knife or mandolin

1 large carrot, peeled and julienned

½ medium   white onion, thinly sliced

Dressing:

3 tablespoons aquafaba (chickpea cooking liquid)

½ cup canola oil

1 tablespoon apple cider vinegar

2 tablespoons lemon juice

2 tablespoons honey

½ teaspoon sea salt, or more to taste

Directions:

Combine the vegetables in a bowl. In a blender, add the aquafaba and slowly drizzle in the oil. Add the remaining dressing ingredients and blend. Pour this dressing over the vegetables and toss to combine. Taste and add salt.

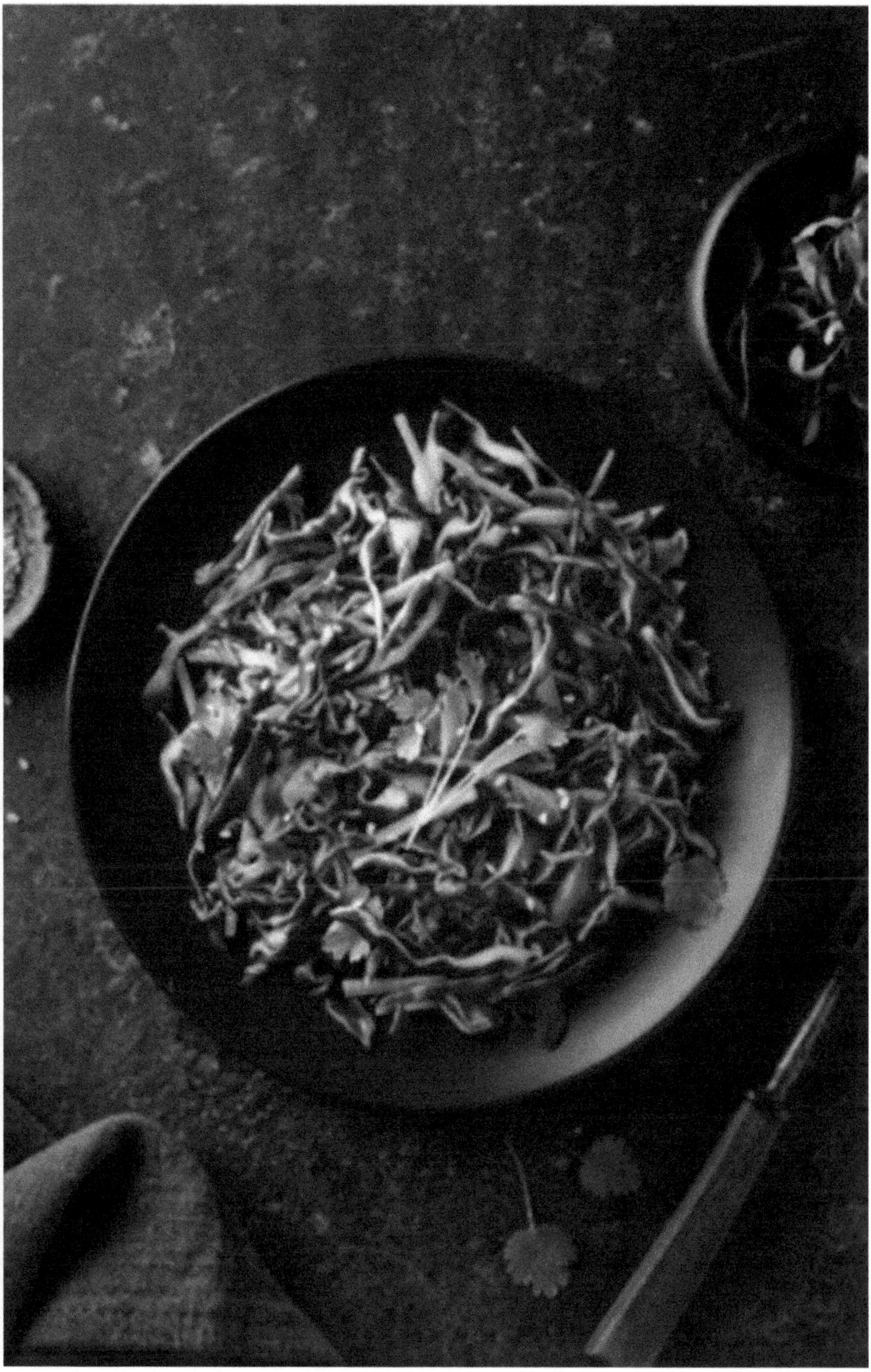

Vegetarian Macaroni and Cheese

Ingredients

3 1/2 cups elbow macaroni

1/2 cup butter

1/2 cup flour

3 1/2 cups boiling water

1-2 tsp. sea salt

2 Tbsp. soy sauce

1 1/2 tsp. garlic powder

Pinch of turmeric

1/4 cup olive oil

1 cup nutritional yeast flakes Spanish Paprika, to taste

Directions:

Preheat your oven to 350°F. Cook the elbow macaroni according to the package instructions. Drain the noodles. In a pan, heat the vegan margarine on low until melted. Add and whisk the flour. Continue whisking and increase to medium heat until smooth and bubbly. Add and whisk in the boiling water, salt, soy sauce, garlic powder, and turmeric. Continue to whisk until dissolved. Once thick and bubbly, whisk in the oil and the yeast flakes. Mix 3/4 of the sauce with the noodles and place in a baking dish. Pour the remaining sauce and season with the paprika. Bake for 15 minutes. Broil until crisp for a few min.

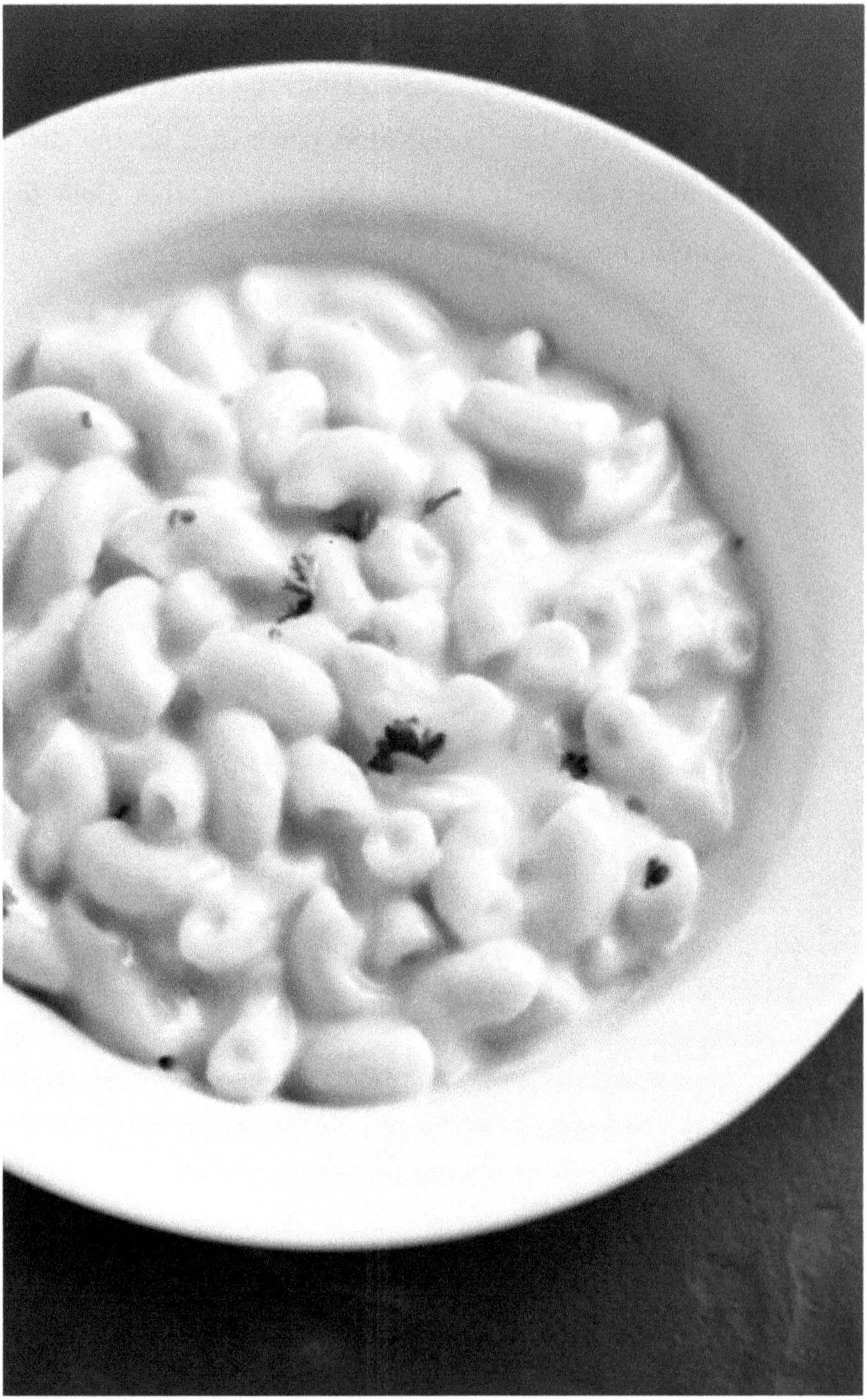

Vegetarian Pizza

Ingredients

1 piece vegan naan (Indian flatbread)

2 Tbsp. tomato sauce

1/4 cup shredded mozzarella

1/4 cup chopped fresh button mushrooms

3 thin tomato slices

2 vegan meatballs Quorn, thawed (if frozen) and cut into small pieces

1 tsp. vegan Parmesan

Pinch of dried basil

Pinch of dried oregano

½ tsp. sea salt

Directions:

Preheat your oven to 350°F. Place the naan on a baking pan. Layer the sauce evenly over the top and sprinkle with half the vegan mozzarella shreds. Add in the mushrooms, tomato slices, and vegan meatball pieces. Layer with the rest of the vegan mozzarella shreds. Lightly season with the vegan Parmesan, basil, and oregano. Bake for 25 minutes.

Tofu Stir Fry

Ingredients

1 package firm tofu, drained and mashed

Juice of 1/2 lemon

1/2 tsp. salt

1/2 tsp. turmeric

1 Tbsp. extra virgin olive oil

1/4 cup diced jalapeno

1/4 cup diced red onion

3 clove garlic, minced

1 Tbsp. chopped flat-leaf parsley

1 Tbsp. vegan bacon bits (optional)

Pepper, to taste (optional)

Directions:

In a bowl, mix the crumbled tofu, lemon juice, salt, and turmeric thoroughly. Heat the oil over medium heat and add the jalapeno, onion, and garlic. Stir fry for 2 1/2 minutes, or until just softened. Add the tofu mixture and cook for 15 minutes. Garnish with parsley, soy bacon pieces, and pepper.

Simple Watercress Stir Fry

Ingredients

1 package firm watercress, rinsed and drained

Juice of 1/2 lemon

1/2 tsp. salt

1 Tbsp. extra virgin olive oil

1/4 cup diced green pepper

1/4 cup diced red onion

3 clove garlic, minced

1 Tbsp. chopped flat-leaf parsley

1 Tbsp. vegan bacon bits (optional)

Pepper, to taste (optional)

Directions:

In a bowl, mix the watercress, lemon juice, & salt thoroughly. Heat the oil over medium heat and add the pepper, onion, and garlic. Stir fry for 2 1/2 minutes, or until just softened. Add the tofu mixture and cook for 15 minutes. Garnish with parsley, soy bacon pieces, and pepper.

Simple Bok Choy Stir Fry

Ingredients

1 bunch bok choy, rinsed and drained

1/2 tsp. salt

1/2 tsp. Chinese chili garlic paste

1 Tbsp. sesame oil

1/4 cup diced green pepper

1/4 cup diced red onion

3 clove garlic, minced

1 Tbsp. chopped flat-leaf parsley

1 Tbsp. vegan bacon bits (optional)

Pepper, to taste (optional)

Directions:

In a bowl, mix the bok choy, chili garlic paste & salt thoroughly. Heat the oil over medium heat and add the pepper, onion, and garlic. Stir fry for 2 1/2 minutes, or until just softened. Add the tofu mixture and cook for 15 minutes. Garnish with parsley, soy bacon pieces, and pepper.

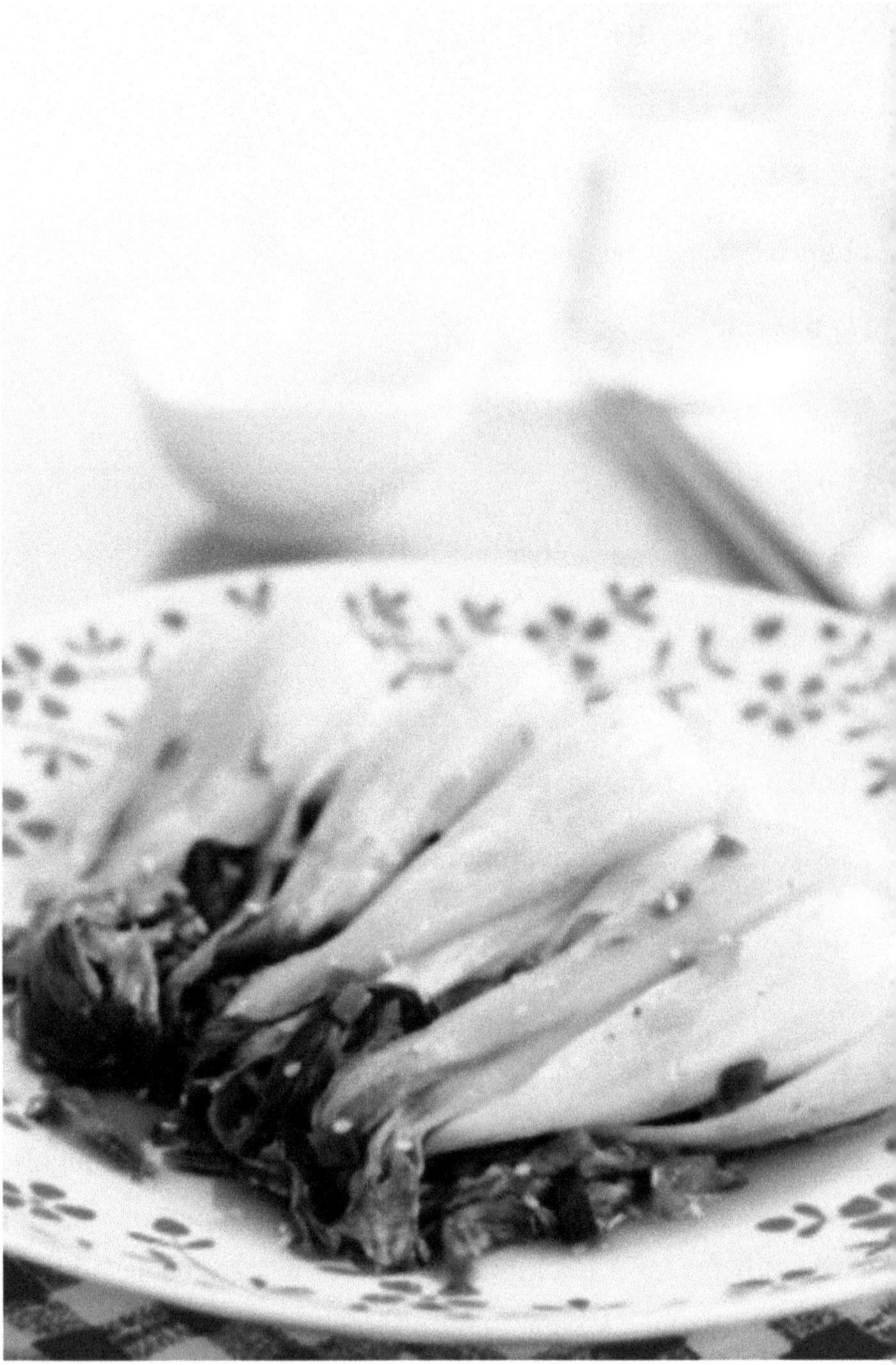

Easy Broccoli Stir Fry

Ingredients

20 pcs. broccoli, rinsed, rinsed, and drained

Juice of 1/2 lemon

1/2 tsp. salt

1 Tbsp. extra virgin olive oil

1/4 cup diced green pepper

1/4 cup diced red onion

3 clove garlic, minced

1 Tbsp. chopped flat-leaf parsley

1 Tbsp. vegan bacon bits (optional)

Pepper, to taste (optional)

In a bowl, mix the broccoli, lemon juice, and salt thoroughly.

Directions:

Heat the oil over medium heat and add the pepper, onion, and garlic. Stir fry for 2 1/2 minutes, or until just softened. Add the tofu mixture and cook for 15 minutes. Garnish with parsley, soy bacon pieces, and pepper.

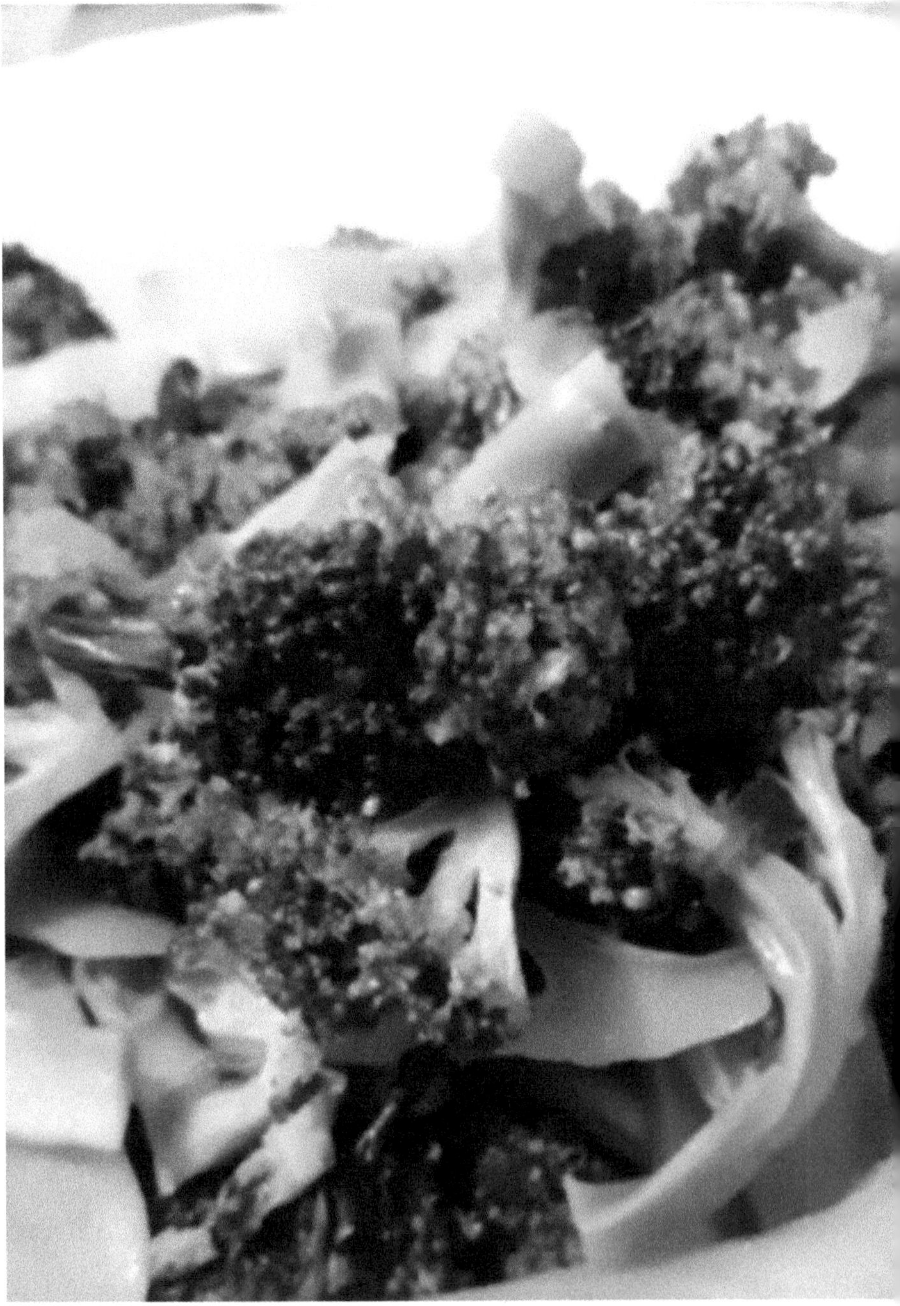

Vegetarian Alfredo Sauce

Ingredients

1/4 cup butter

3 cloves garlic, minced

2 cups cooked white beans, rinsed and drained

1 1/2 cups unsweetened almond milk

Sea salt and pepper, to taste

Parsley (optional)

Directions:

Melt the butter on low heat. Add the garlic and cook for 2 ½ minutes. Transfer to a food processor, add the beans and 1 cup of almond milk. Blend until smooth. Pour the sauce into the pan over low heat and season with salt and pepper. Add the parsley. Cook until warm.

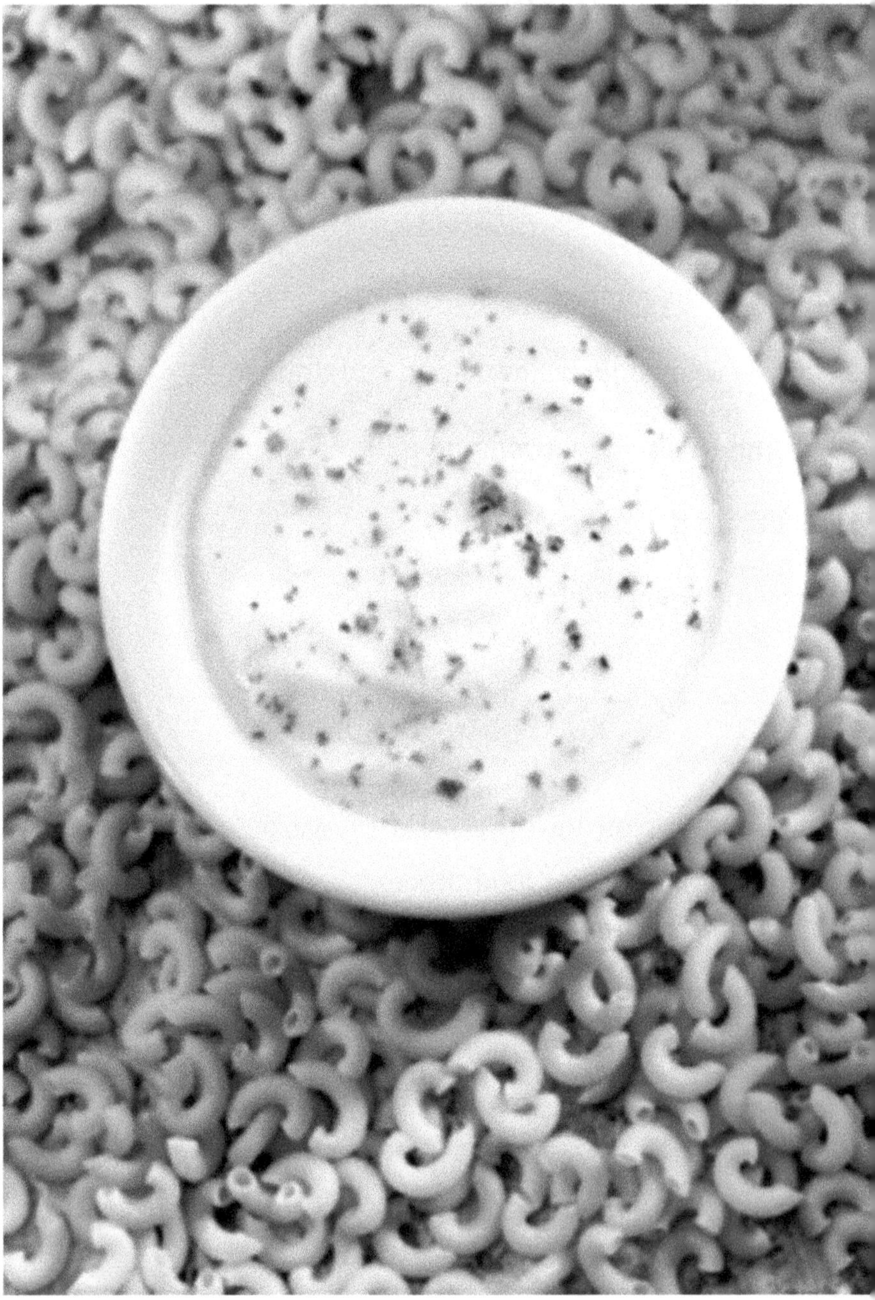

Vegan Fajitas

Ingredients

1 can Refried Beans (15oz)

1 can Lima Beans (15oz), drained and rinsed

1/4 cup Salsa

1 Red Onion sliced into strips

1 Green Bell Pepper sliced into strips

2 Tbsp Lime Juice

2 tsp Fajita Spice Mix (see below) Tortillas Fajita Mix

1 Tbsp. Corn Starch

2 tsp Chili Powder

1 tsp Spanish Paprika

1 tsp honey

1/2 tsp Sea salt

1/2 teaspoon Onion Powder

1/2 teaspoon Garlic Powder

1/2 teaspoon Ground Cumin

1/8 teaspoon Cayenne Pepper

Directions:

Simmer salsa and refried beans until warm. Add and mix the fajita) mix ingredients in a small bowl and leave 2 tsp. Behind. Sauté the onion, pepper, and 2 tsp of Spice Mix in water and lime juice. Continue until liquid evaporates and vegetables start to brown Layer the beans in the middle of the tortilla. Layer with the stir-fried veggies and toppings. Roll it up and serve.

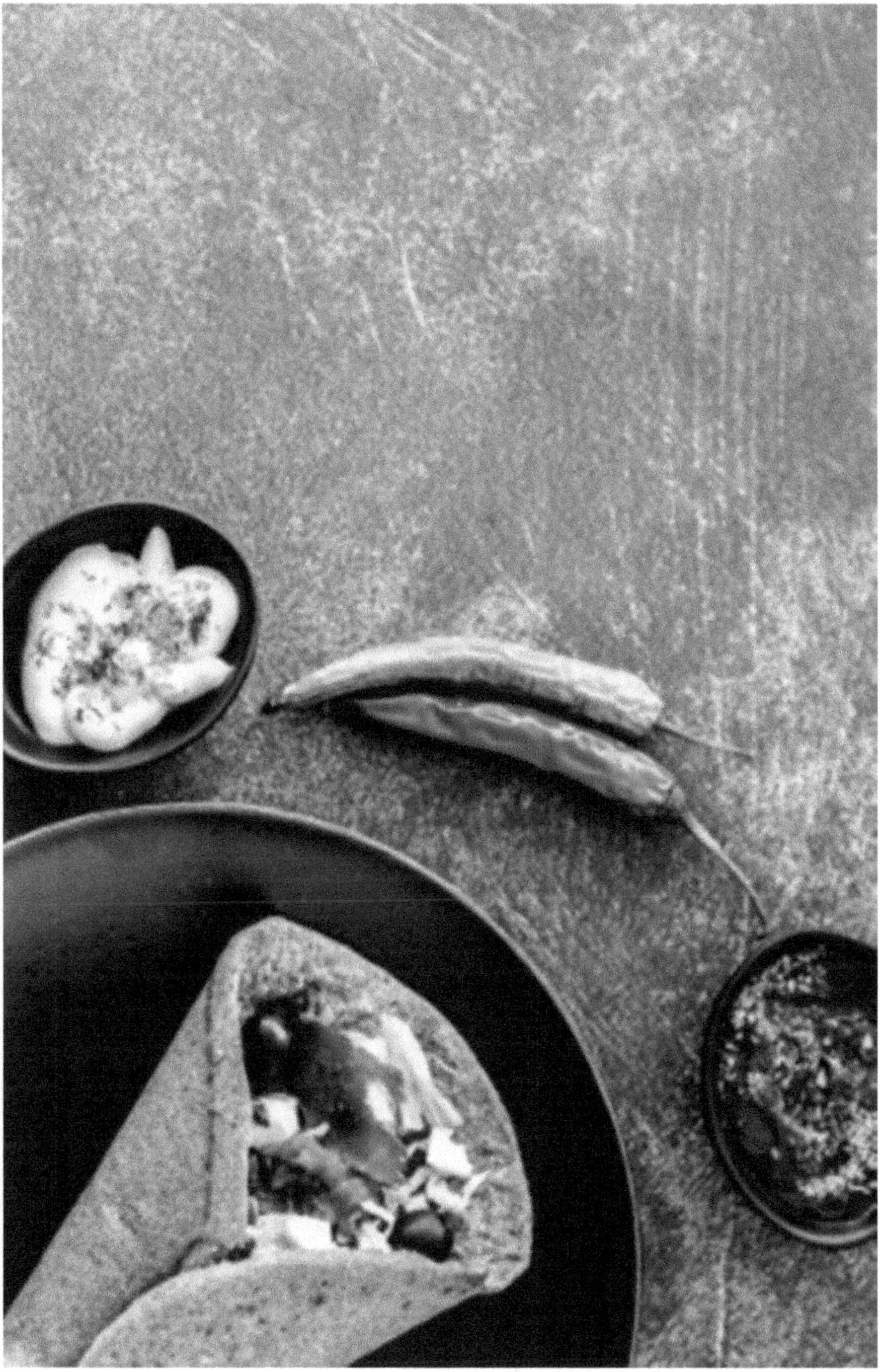

Grilled Summer Squash and Zucchini

Ingredients

1 summer squash, peeled and sliced lengthwise

1 lb zucchini, sliced lengthwise into shorter sticks

1 lb yellow bell peppers, sliced into wide strips

10 Broccolini Florets

10 pcs. Brussel Sprouts

1 large red onion, cut into 1/2 inch thick rounds

1/3 cup Italian parsley or basil, finely chopped

Dressing:

6 tbsp. extra virgin olive oil

Sea salt, to taste

3 tbsp. apple cider vinegar

1 tbsp. honey

Directions:

Egg-free mayonnaise Combine all of the dressing ingredients thoroughly. Preheat your grill to low heat and grease the grates.

Layer the vegetable grill for 12 minutes per side until tender, flipping once. Brush with the marinade/ dressing ingredients

Grilled Beetroots and Artichoke Hearts

Ingredients

1 cup artichoke hearts

2 beetroots, peeled and sliced lengthwise

1 large red onion, cut into 1/2 inch thick rounds

1/3 cup Italian parsley or basil, finely chopped

Dressing:

6 tbsp. extra virgin olive oil

Sea salt, to taste

3 tbsp. apple cider vinegar

1 tbsp. honey

Directions:

Egg-free mayonnaise Combine all of the dressing ingredients thoroughly. Preheat your grill to low heat and grease the grates. Layer the vegetable grill for 12 minutes per side until tender, flipping once. Brush with the marinade/ dressing ingredients

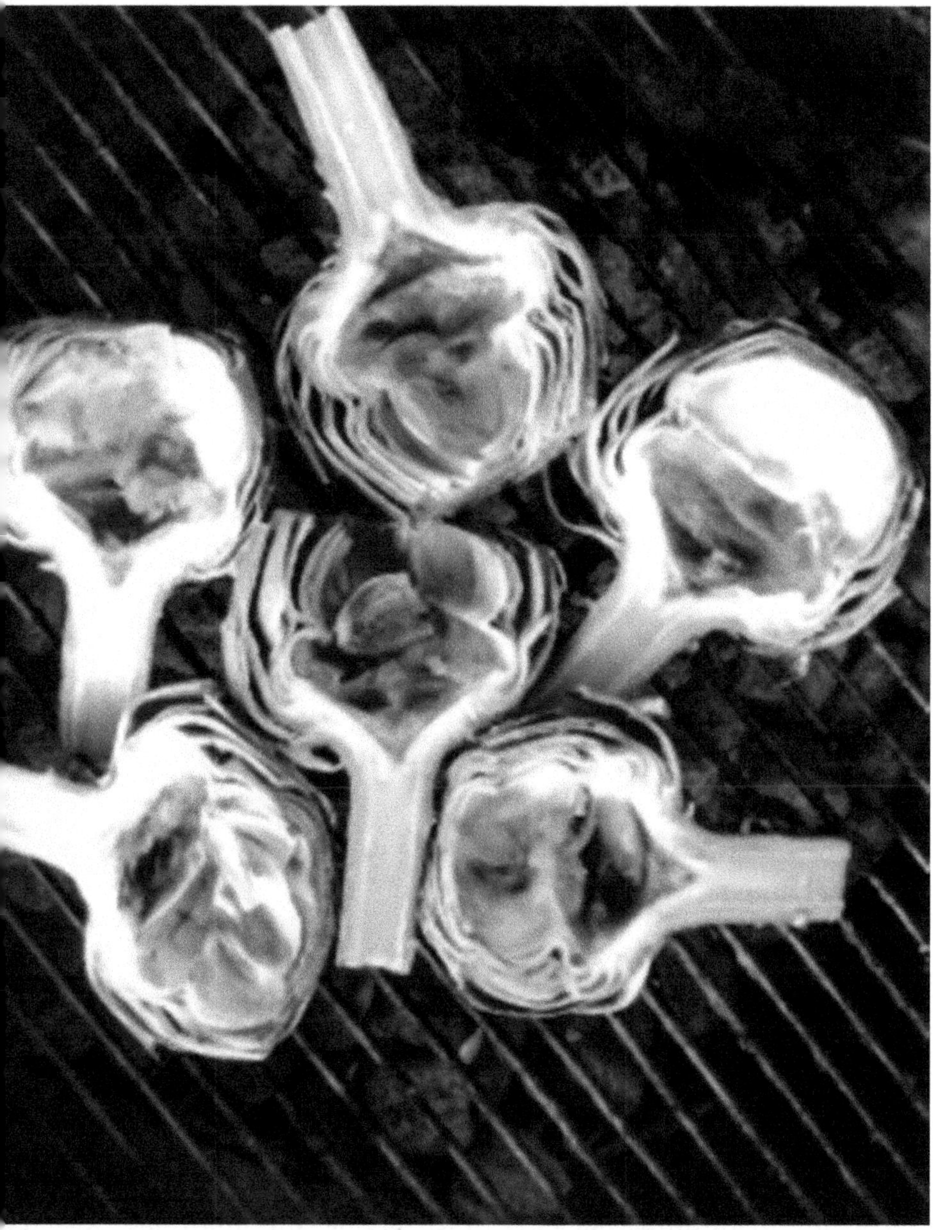

Grilled Cabbage and Collard Greens

Ingredients

1 medium Cabbage sliced

1 bunch of collard greens

1 large red onion, cut into 1/2 inch thick rounds

1/3 cup Italian parsley or basil, finely chopped

Dressing Ingredients

6 tbsp. olive oil

1 tsp. garlic powder

1 tsp. onion powder

Sea salt, to taste

3 tbsp. white wine vinegar

English mustard

Directions:

Combine all of the dressing ingredients thoroughly. Preheat your grill to low heat and grease the grates. Layer the vegetable grill for 12 minutes per side until tender, flipping once. Brush with the marinade/ dressing ingredients

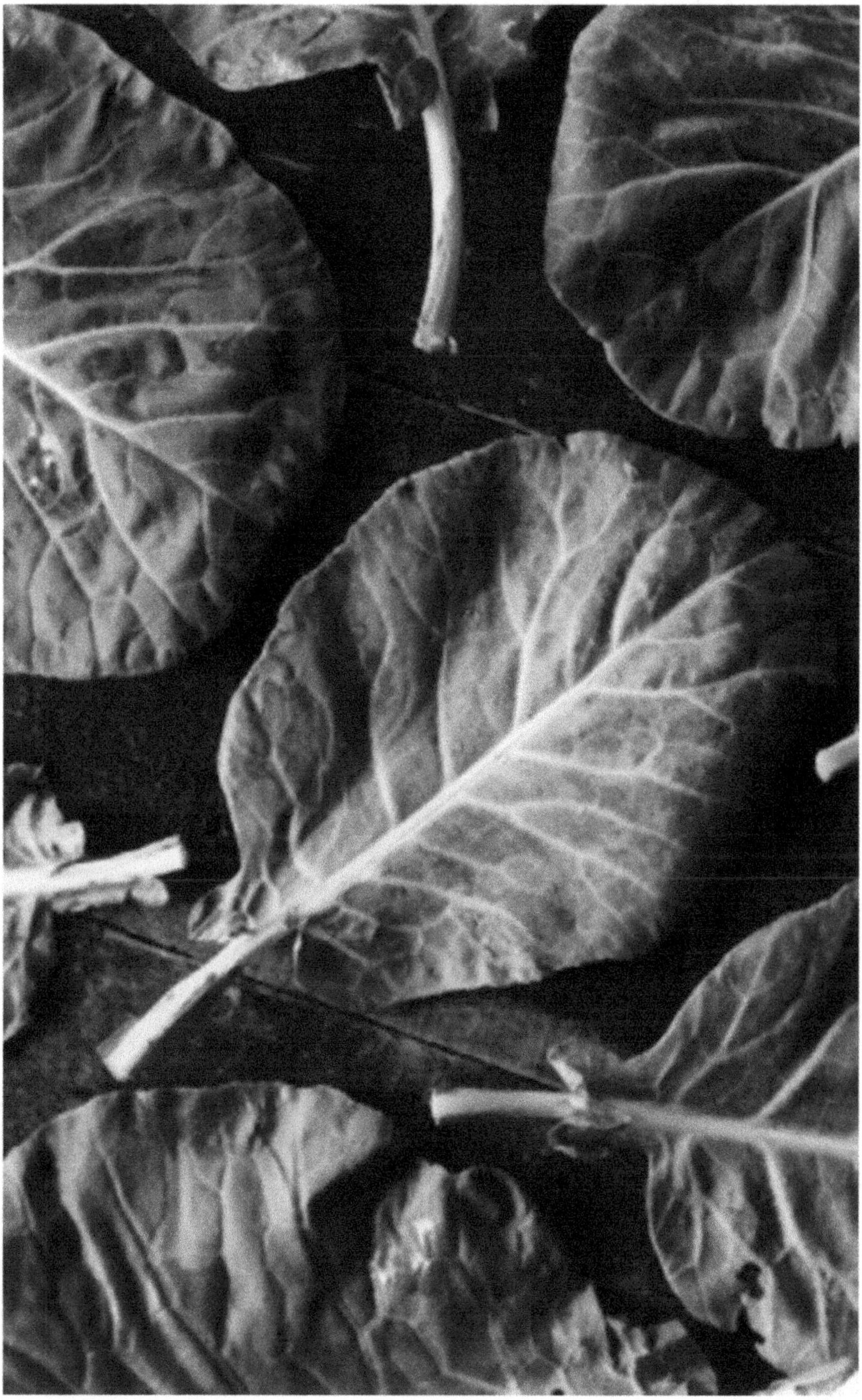

Grilled Artichoke and Mustard Greens

Ingredients

1 pc. Artichoke

1 bunch of mustard greens

2 medium carrots, cut lengthwise and cut in half

4 large Tomatoes, sliced thick

Dressing:

6 tbsp. extra virgin olive oil

Sea salt, to taste

3 tbsp. Balsamic vinegar

Directions:

Dijon mustard Combine all of the dressing ingredients thoroughly. Preheat your grill to low heat and grease the grates. Layer the vegetable grill for 12 minutes per side until tender, flipping once. Brush with the marinade/ dressing ingredients

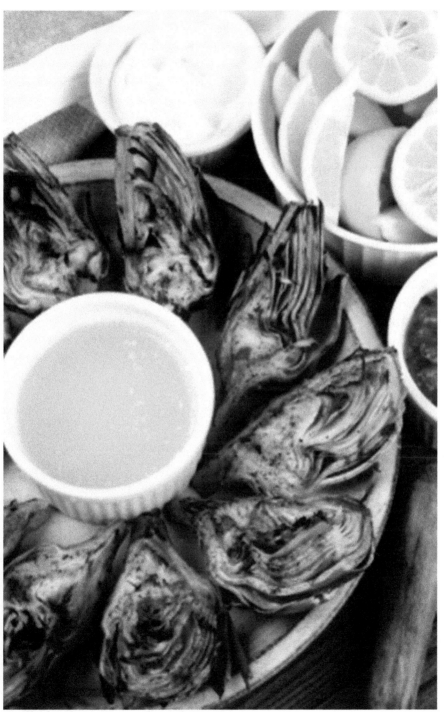

Grilled Winter Squash and Beets

Ingredients

5 pcs. Beets

1 winter squash, peeled and sliced lengthwise

10 pcs. Brussel Sprouts

1 large red onion, cut into

1/2 inch thick rounds

1/3 cup Italian parsley or basil, finely chopped

Dressing:

6 tbsp. extra virgin olive oil

Sea salt, to taste

3 tbsp. apple cider vinegar

1 tbsp. honey

Directions:

Egg-free mayonnaise Combine all of the dressing ingredients thoroughly. Preheat your grill to low heat and grease the grates. Layer the vegetable grill for 12 minutes per side until tender, flipping once. Brush with the marinade/ dressing ingredients

Grilled Cabbage and Mustard Greens

Ingredients

1 medium Cabbage sliced

1 bunch of mustard greens

1/3 cup Italian parsley or basil, finely chopped

Dressing:

6 tbsp. extra virgin olive oil

Sea salt, to taste

3 tbsp. Balsamic vinegar

Directions:

Combine all of the dressing ingredients thoroughly. Preheat your grill to low heat and grease the grates. Layer the vegetable grill for 12 minutes per side until tender, flipping once. Brush with the marinade/ dressing ingredients

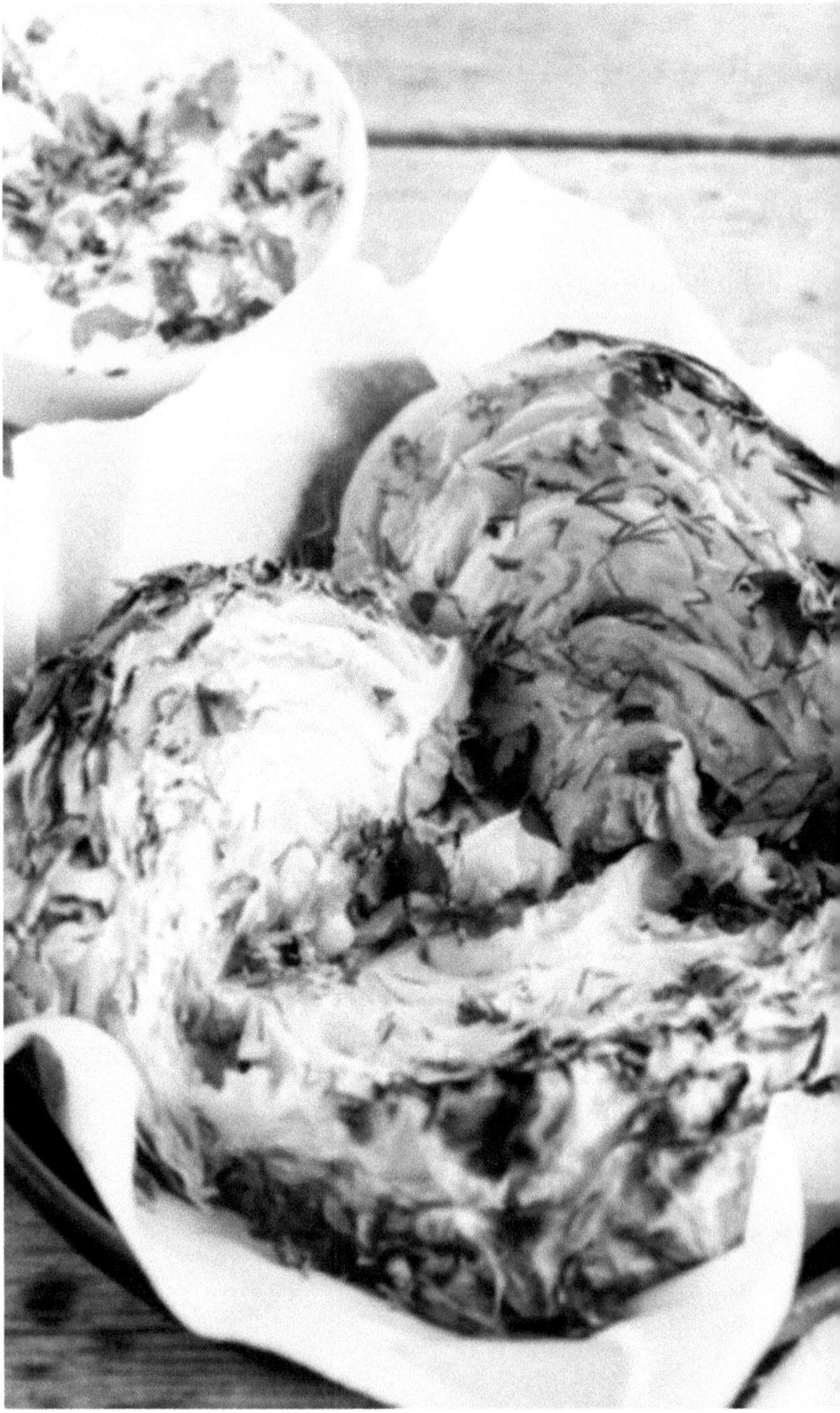

Grilled Okra and Red Onions

Ingredients

10 pcs. Okra

1 large red onion, cut into

1/2 inch thick rounds

1/3 cup Italian parsley or basil, finely chopped

Dressing:

6 tbsp. olive oil

1 tsp. garlic powder

1 tsp. onion powder

Sea salt, to taste

3 tbsp. white wine vinegar

Directions:

English mustard Combine all of the dressing ingredients thoroughly. Preheat your grill to low heat and grease the grates. Layer the vegetable grill for 12 minutes per side until tender, flipping once. Brush with the marinade/ dressing ingredients

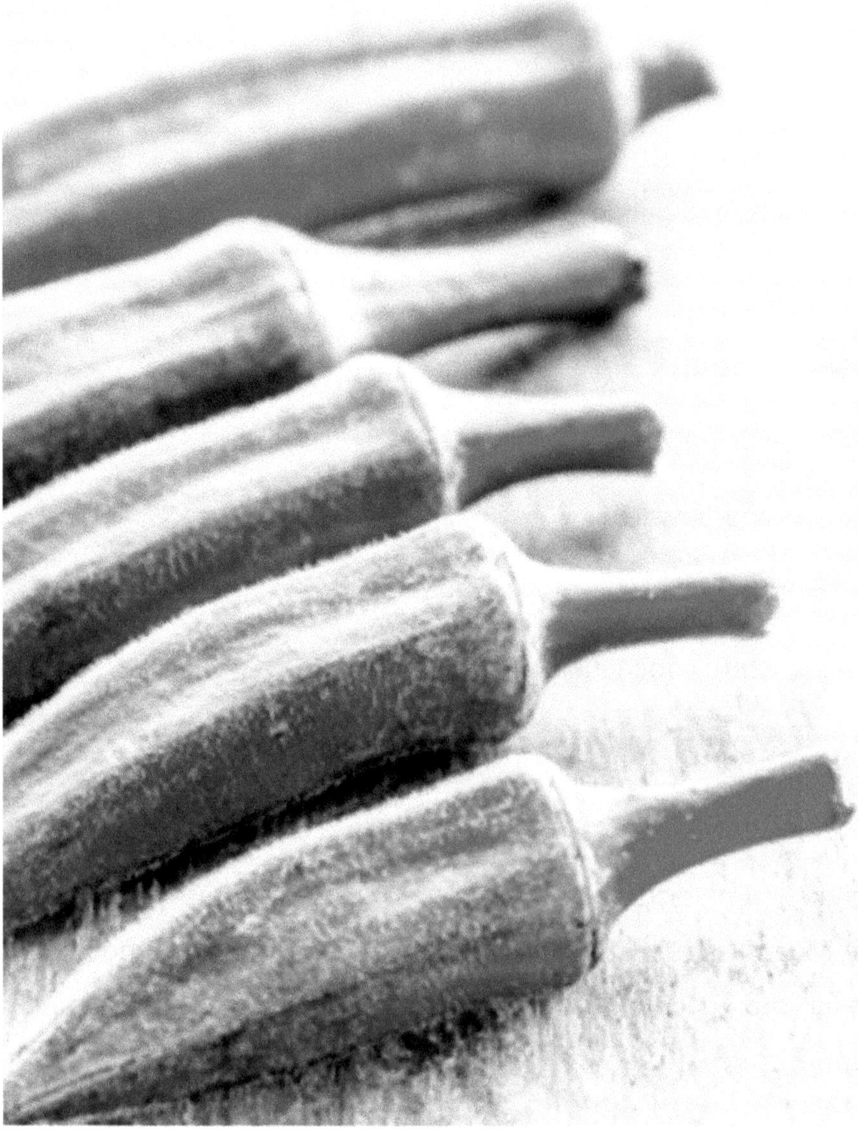

Grilled Kale and Romaine Lettuce

Ingredients

1 bunch of Kale

1 bunch of Romaine Lettuce leaves

1 winter squash, peeled and sliced lengthwise

1/3 cup Italian parsley or basil, finely chopped

Dressing:

6 tbsp. extra virgin olive oil

Sea salt, to taste

3 tbsp. Balsamic vinegar

Directions:

Dijon mustard Combine all of the dressing ingredients thoroughly. Preheat your grill to low heat and grease the grates. Layer the vegetable grill for 12 minutes per side until tender, flipping once. Brush with the marinade/ dressing ingredients

Grilled Okra and Endives

Ingredients

10 pcs. Okra

1 bunch of endives

1/3 cup Italian parsley or basil, finely chopped

Dressing:

6 tbsp. olive oil

3 dashes of Tabasco hot sauce

Sea salt, to taste

3 tbsp. white wine vinegar

Directions:

Egg-free mayonnaise Combine all of the dressing ingredients thoroughly. Preheat your grill to low heat and grease the grates. Layer the vegetable grill for 12 minutes per side until tender, flipping once. Brush with the marinade/ dressing ingredients

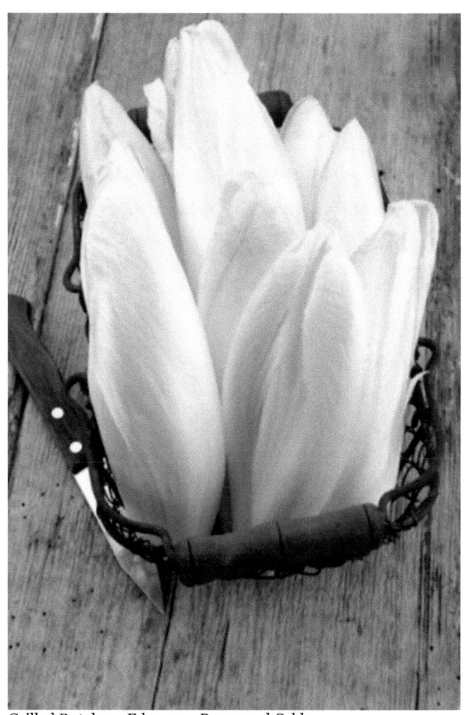

Grilled Rutabaga Edamame Beans and Cabbage

Ingredients

20 pcs. Edamame Beans

1 medium Cabbage sliced

1 medium Rutabaga, peeled and cut in half lengthwise

2 medium carrots, cut lengthwise and cut in half

4 large Tomatoes, sliced thick

1/3 cup Italian parsley or basil, finely chopped

Dressing:

6 tbsp. olive oil

3 dashes of Tabasco hot sauce

Sea salt, to taste

3 tbsp. white wine vinegar

Directions:

Egg-free mayonnaise Combine all of the dressing ingredients thoroughly. Preheat your grill to low heat and grease the grates. Layer the vegetable grill for 12 minutes per side until tender, flipping once. Brush with the marinade/ dressing ingredients

Grilled Summer Squash Beets and Artichoke Hearts

Ingredients

5 pcs. Beets 1 cup artichoke hearts

1 bunch of Romaine Lettuce leaves

1 butternut squash, peeled and sliced lengthwise

4 large Tomatoes, sliced thick

Dressing:

6 tbsp. olive oil

3 dashes of Tabasco hot sauce

Sea salt, to taste

3 tbsp. white wine vinegar

Directions:

Egg-free mayonnaise Combine all of the dressing ingredients thoroughly. Preheat your grill to low heat and grease the grates. Layer the vegetable grill for 12 minutes per side until tender, flipping once. Brush with the marinade/ dressing ingredients

Grilled Button and Shitake Mushroom

Ingredients

12 oz. fresh button mushrooms

4 oz. shiitake mushrooms

1 bunch of collard greens

4 tablespoons canola oil, divided

Sea salt and freshly ground black pepper

2 tablespoons reduced-sodium soy sauce

2 tablespoons unseasoned rice vinegar

1 tablespoon toasted sesame oil

1 teaspoon finely grated peeled ginger

6 scallions, thinly sliced on a diagonal

2 teaspoons toasted sesame seeds

Directions:

Combine the mushrooms and carrots with 3 Tbsp. Canola oil in a bowl. Season with salt and pepper. Grill while turning the mushrooms and carrots frequently until tender. Combine the soy sauce, vinegar, sesame oil, ginger, and remaining 1 Tbsp.

Canola oil in a bowl. Cut the carrots into 2 inch long pieces. Cut the mushrooms into bite-size pieces. Combine them with the vinaigrette, scallions, and sesame seeds. Season with salt and pepper.

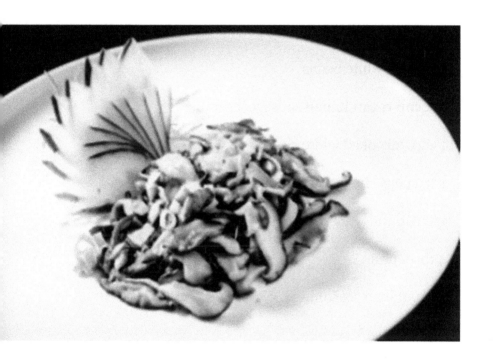

White Beans and Italian Sausage Burrito Bowl

Ingredients

1 red onion, diced or thinly sliced

1 green bell pepper (I used yellow), diced

1 mild red chili, finely chopped

1 1/2 cup white beans

1/2 cup vegan Italian sausage, crumbled

1 cup uncooked white rice

1 1/2 cups chopped tomatoes

1/2 cup water

4 tbsp. pesto

1 tsp. Italian seasoning

Sea salt Black pepper

Toppings: fresh coriander (cilantro), chopped spring onions, sliced avocado, guacamole, etc.

Directions:

Combine all the burrito bowl ingredients (not toppings) in a slow cooker. Cook on low for 3 hours, or until the rice is cooked. Serve hot with topping ingredients

Smoky Red Rice with Garbanzo Beans

Ingredients

1 poblano chili, diced

1 red onion, diced

1 mild red chili, finely chopped

1/2 cup vegan burger (Brand: Beyond Meat Beyond Burger), crumbled

1 ½ cups garbanzo beans, drained

1 cup uncooked red rice

1 ½ cups chopped tomatoes

½ cup water

4 tbsp. chimichurri sauce

1/2 tsp. cayenne pepper

Sea salt Black pepper

Toppings: fresh coriander (cilantro), chopped spring onions, sliced avocado, guacamole, etc.

Directions:

Combine all the burrito bowl ingredients (not toppings) in a slow cooker. Cook on low for 3 hours, or until the rice is cooked. Serve hot with topping ingredients

Vegan Chorizo Burrito Bowl

Ingredients

1 ancho chili, diced

1 red onion, diced

1 mild red chili, finely chopped

1/2 cup vegan Chorizo (Soyrizo), crumbled

1 cup uncooked white rice

1 1/2 cups chopped tomatoes

1/2 cup water

1/4 cup vegan chorizos, coarsely chopped

1 tsp. dried thyme

Sea salt Black pepper

Toppings: fresh coriander (cilantro), chopped spring onions, sliced avocado, guacamole, etc.

Directions:

Combine all the burrito bowl ingredients (not toppings) in a slow cooker. Cook on low for 3 hours, or until the rice is cooked. Serve hot with topping ingredients

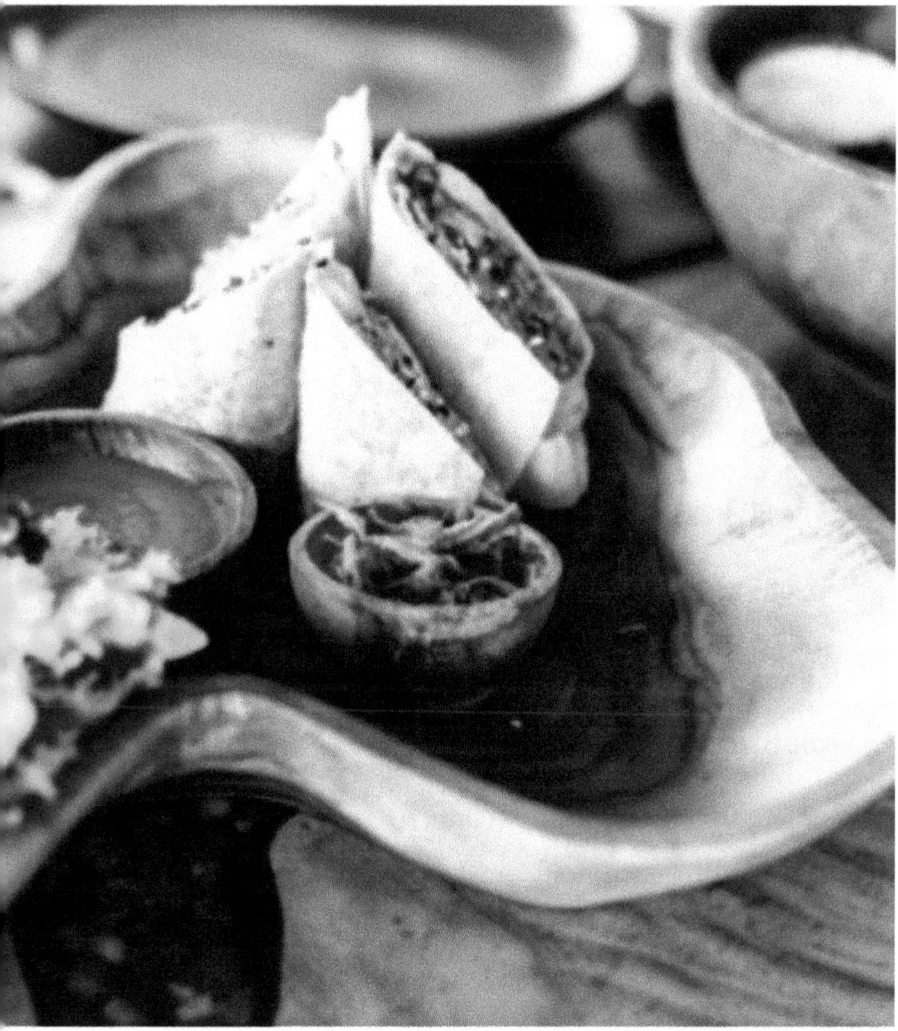

Chimichurri Vegan Chorizo Burrito Bowl

Ingredients

1 Anaheim pepper, diced

1 red onion, diced

1 mild red chili, finely chopped

1/2 cup vegan Chorizo (Soyrizo), crumbled

1 cup uncooked red rice

1 ½ cups chopped tomatoes

½ cup water

4 tbsp. chimichurri sauce

1/2 tsp. cayenne pepper

Sea salt Black pepper

Toppings: fresh coriander (cilantro), chopped spring onions, sliced avocado, guacamole, etc.

Directions:

Combine all the burrito bowl ingredients (not toppings) in a slow cooker. Cook on low for 3 hours, or until the rice is cooked. Serve hot with topping ingredients

Smoky White Bean & White Rice Burrito Bowl

Ingredients

1 red onion, diced or thinly sliced

1/2 cup meatless meatballs, crumbled

1 mild red chili, finely chopped

1 1/2 cup white beans

1 cup uncooked white rice

1 1/2 cups chopped tomatoes

1/2 cup water

1 tbsp chipotle hot sauce (or other favorite hot sauce)

1 tsp smoked paprika

1/2 tsp ground cumin

Sea salt Black pepper

Toppings: fresh coriander (cilantro), chopped spring onions, sliced avocado, guacamole, etc.

Directions:

Combine all the burrito bowl ingredients (not toppings) in a slow cooker. Cook on low for 3 hours, or until the rice is cooked. Serve hot with topping ingredients

Red Rice with Vegan Chorizo and Tomatoes

Ingredients

1 poblano chili, diced

1 red onion, diced

1/2 cup vegan Chorizo (Soyrizo), crumbled

1 ½ cups garbanzo beans, drained

1 cup uncooked red rice

1 ½ cups chopped tomatoes

½ cup water

4 tbsp. chimichurri sauce

1/2 tsp. cayenne pepper

Sea salt Black pepper

Toppings: fresh coriander (cilantro), chopped spring onions, sliced avocado, guacamole, etc.

Directions:

Combine all the burrito bowl ingredients (not toppings) in a slow cooker. Cook on low for 3 hours, or until the rice is cooked. Serve hot with topping ingredients

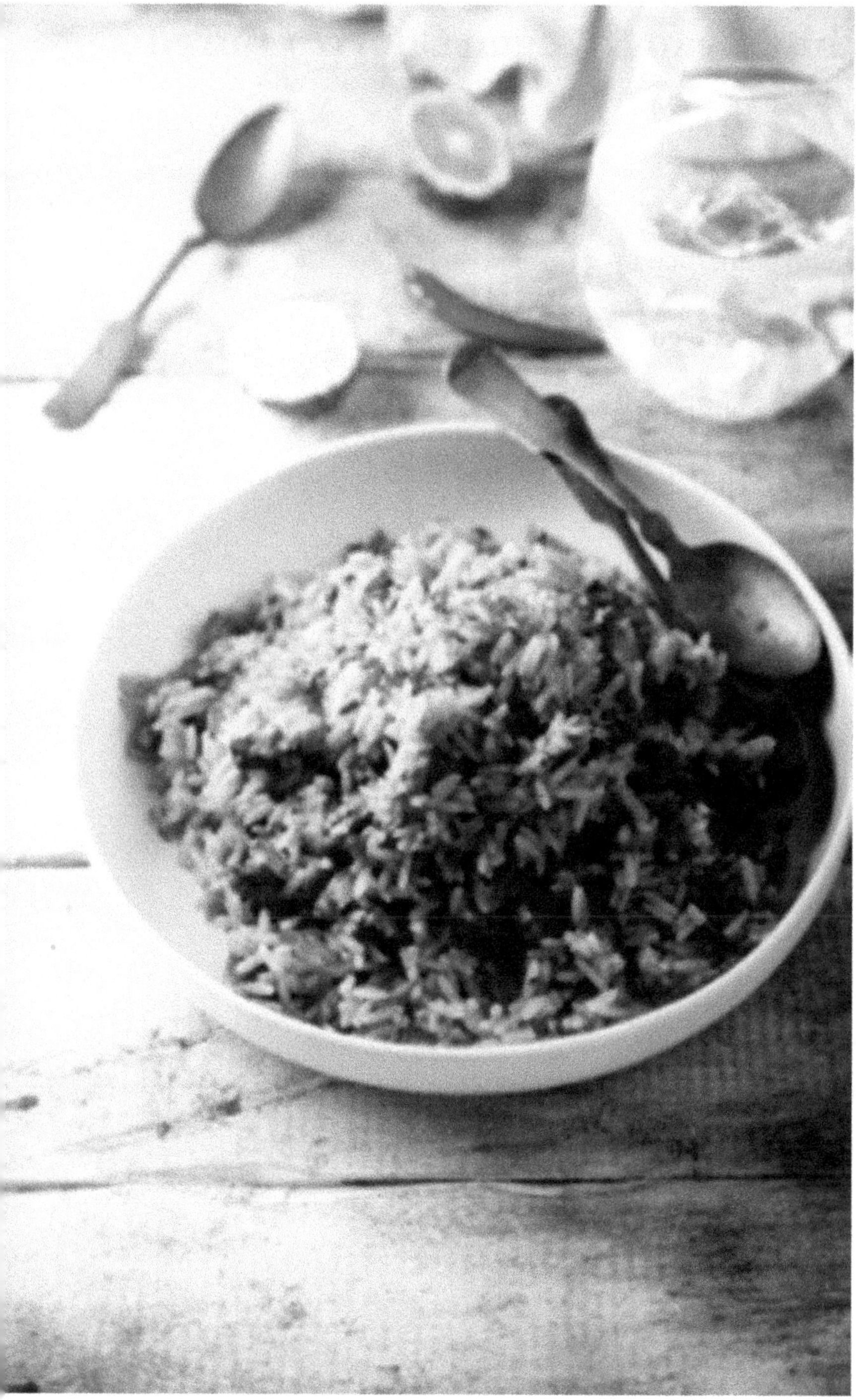

White Bean & Vegan Chorizo Burrito

Ingredients

1 ancho chili, diced

1 red onion, diced

1 mild red chili, finely chopped

1 1/2 cup white beans

1 cup uncooked white rice

1 1/2 cups chopped tomatoes

1/2 cup water

1/4 cup vegan chorizos, coarsely chopped

1/2 cup meatless meatballs, crumbled

1 tsp. dried thyme

Sea salt Black pepper

Toppings: fresh coriander (cilantro), chopped spring onions, sliced avocado, guacamole, etc.

Directions:

Combine all the burrito bowl ingredients (not toppings) in a slow cooker. Cook on low for 3 hours, or until the rice is cooked. Serve hot with topping ingredients

Parmesan Cauliflower Steak

Servings: 4 Servings

Ingredients

1 large head cauliflower 4 tbsp butter

2 tbsp Urban Accents Manchego and Roasted Garlic seasoning blend

1/4 cup parmesan cheese Salt and pepper to taste

Instructions

Preheat oven to 400 degrees Remove leaves from cauliflower Slice cauliflower lengthwise through core into 1 inch steaks (mine made about 4) Melt butter in microwave and mix with seasoning blend to make paste

Brush mixture over steaks and season with salt and pepper to taste Heat non-stick pan over medium and place cauliflower steaks for 2-3 minutes until lightly browned Flip carefully, repeat. Place cauliflower steaks on lined baking sheet. Bake cauliflower steaks in oven for 15-20 minutes until golden and tender. Sprinkle with parmesan cheese and serve.

Vegetarian Red Coconut Curry

Servingss 2 servings

Ingredients

1 cup broccoli florets

1 large handful of spinach 4 tablespoons coconut oil

¼ medium onion

1 teaspoon minced garlic 1 teaspoon minced ginger

2 teaspoons Fysh sauce

2 teaspoons soy sauce

1 tablespoon red curry paste

½ cup coconut cream (or coconut milk)

Instructions

Add 2 tbsp. coconut oil to a pan and bring to medium-high heat.

Chop onions and mince garlic while you wait. When the oil is hot, add the onion to the pan and let it sizzle. Allow it to cook for 3-4 minutes to caramelize and become semi-translucent. Once this happens, add the garlic to the pan and let it brown slightly. About 30 seconds.

Turn the heat to medium-low and add broccoli florets to the pan. aStir everything together well. Let the broccoli take on the flavors of the onion and garlic. This should take about 1-2 minutes. Move everything in your pan to the side and add 1 tbsp. red curry paste. You want this hitting the bottom of the pan so that all of the flavors can be released from the spices. Once your red curry paste starts to smell pungent, mix everything together again and add a large handful of spinach over the top. Once the spinach begins to wilt, add coconut cream and mix together. Stir everything together and then add 2 tbsp. more coconut oil, 2 tsp. fysh sauce, 2 tsp. soy sauce, and 1 tsp. minced ginger. Let this simmer for 5-10 minutes, depending on how thick you want the sauce. Dish out and serve! Feel free to garnish with a few slices of red cabbage and black sesame seeds for color.

Nutrition Info

398 Calories 40.73g Fats 7.86g Carbs

Lightning Source UK Ltd.
Milton Keynes UK
UKHW020750230421
382488UK00001B/33